Get a

GOLD
MEDAL
BUTT

Get a
GOLD MEDAL BUTT

Gary Guerriero
and
Mary Leonard
with Ron Holland

Photos by Tim Dalal
Modeling by Olympian Fencer Sharon Monplaisir

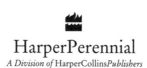

HarperPerennial
A Division of HarperCollinsPublishers

As with any new diet or exercise regimen, readers are strongly encouraged to consult with a physician before attempting to embark on any of the programs or procedures contained in this book. While every care has been taken to ensure that the contents are accurate, the authors and the publisher cannot accept legal responsibility for any problems arising from the use of the methods and information described in this book.

ISBN 0-06-095190-7

96 97 98 99 00 ❖/RRD 10 9 8 7 6 5 4 3 2 1

CONTENTS

Foreword by Peter Westbrook   vii
Acknowledgments   ix
Introduction   xi

ONE
The Basics   1

TWO
The Gold Medal Fat-Buster Plan   19

THREE
The Newly Active Lifestyle   37

FOUR
Ready, Set, Go!   41

FIVE
Month One   47

SIX
Month Two   65

SEVEN
Month Three   81

EIGHT
Gold Medal Butt Optionals   103

NINE
Beyond the Home Program   113

TEN
Special Trunk and Abdominal Strengthening Exercises   147

ELEVEN
Stretches   159

TWELVE
Little Things Mean a Lot   167

THIRTEEN
Questions the Doubting Thomases Ask Mary and Gary   169

FOREWORD

To the Travelers of This Book . . . in Search of Their Gold Medal Butt

My sport is fencing. And I've competed in five Olympiads, winning as America's Bronze Medalist in 1984. In addition, I've been National Champion thirteen times and between 1975 and 1991 I've been a Pan-American Games competitor five times, winning the gold medal in 1983 and the silver in all the others.

Then time caught up with me, my legs gave out, and my career as a competitive fencer was over.

Not so fast.

Because then I met Gary. I told him how my knees were a torture. How my years of fencing had killed my legs. How my dueling days were over. I also told him that I'd heard of his work with professional athletes, of his ability to turn back the calendar, giving them more years to compete. (I didn't tell him of my reaction to such claims back then: "Hogwash!")

Gary began his relentless therapy: prescribing precise moves to strengthen every muscle in my legs, working on me twice each week. Incredibly, but undeniably, his treatments took six full years off my knees. Then, at an ancient age for a fencer, miracles began to happen.

The 1995 Pan-American tryouts: I won!

The Pan-American Games in Argentina: I won the Gold!

The Sabre Team Finals: We won the Gold!

Then I won my unprecedented thirteenth U.S. National Title. Glory be! And now things look great for qualifying for the 1996 Olympics. All because of Gary and Mary and their revolutionary U.S. Athletic Training Center.

I'd like to thank the Wonderful, who sent me Gary and Mary. I'd like to thank *them* for changing the course of time itself. And, of course, I thank them for this book, which is going to beautify the world with more Gold Medal Butts than any other generation has ever seen.

So go ahead. Invest the three months. Like every fencer I've ever known . . . you will soon own your very own Gold Medal Butt.

—*Peter Westbrook*

ACKNOWLEDGMENTS

Our special Gold Medal thanks to

Judith Regan of Regan Books . . . for her loyalty, honesty, and her *patience* in shepherding the two of us all the way through our first book.

And George Lois for his genius, of course, but mostly for never letting us forget The Big Idea!

Dennis Mazzella for doing what no other man can do. In advertising, in design, in riveting surfing stories.

Diane Reverand for being so fair.

Michael Comras for guiding us through the thickets of New York real estate.

To our families, especially Leigh and Patrick.

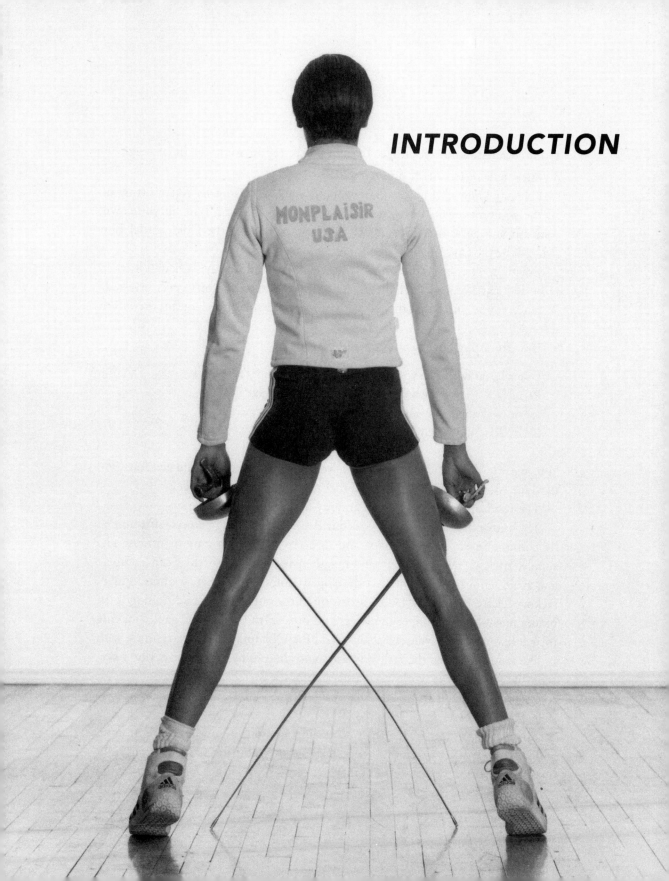

INTRODUCTION

I don't want to know your age. I'm not interested in your weight or height or if you're male or female. It doesn't matter.

I already know all I need to know about you, and here it is: You're sitting on all the equipment you'll ever need to create a Gold Medal Butt all your own. And can you guess how long it will take you to achieve the Gold Medal Butt that will be the envy of your friends (and enemies)?

Exactly 2½ *seconds*. That's how long it will take you to say: "Okay! I'll try it! How do I start?" And they're the most precious 2½ seconds you've ever invested.

Since you've purchased this book, you've passed this step. Got another seven seconds?

If you're sitting down, stand up and do this:

Lean all your weight on your right foot. Tighten your right buttock.
Relax. Now lean all the way to the left. Tighten your left glute.
Relax. Now go up on your toes, and tighten both glutes at once.
Relax. Time's up! You did it!

You just moved it and proved it. You've got all the muscles and tendons you need for your Gold Medal Butt, and they're in good working order.

The rest is up to us three—you and my husband and me.

My husband, Gary, and I spend our days, our working careers, surrounded by bodies of every possible shape and in every imaginable state of fitness: The supple, tireless teenagers that we strengthen for sports—so they can compete and avoid serious injury. The well-developed professional athlete—often injured, seeking release from pain. (And discovering how our unique conditioning techniques makes them stronger than ever and puts them back in the game, making their million-dollar paychecks again.) And the Olympic medalists, training with us like family, to hoist their already awesome abilities by that elusive 4 or 5 percent that separates the world-class athlete from the merely stupendous.

Anyway, in they stream, one physical specimen after another; each enviably skilled and invariably good-natured.

But come into our U.S. Athletic Training Center on any day, look around, and you'll spot a *marvelous* difference. Just as fast and easily as I can; from right up close or from clear across the gym.

In their street clothes or their faded and well-worn workout duds one group stands out, the fencers, bless them all, and for one unmistakable reason: Every last fencer who comes here has a great butt. Young or old, beginners or Olympic medalists, male or female. Round and sound, tight and taut, they *all* have beautiful butts. (Just like the one you're going to have.)

At first, I dismissed the evidence of my own eyes. I mean, it couldn't be a natural law that all fencers had to have a paragon of a posterior. So I looked into it. After all, I'm a trainer, so I can get away with watching people work out. I looked. And *looked*. No question about it.

It's not fair, but it's true: When it comes to rears, fencers have no peers.

So one day I casually opened the subject with Gary.

"Say, Gary. Who do you think has the best butts of anybody in our gym?"

"You mean the fencers?" he said casually.

"Oh, you noticed, too? But how do they get them?"

Gary's curiosity was piqued and, muscle scientist that he is, he grabbed a couple of world champion fencers and studied their movements.

Quick as you could say "touché" we zeroed in on the answer: Six major muscles, engaged through five major movements. You'll soon see, clear as day, how using these muscles and moves can hand you your Gold Medal Butt on a silver platter.

So that's how this book, our program, and *your* Gold Medal Butt was born.

Of course, it didn't happen in a day. These exercises took months to devise, simplify, and test with volunteers. In fact, I insisted on being the first volunteer, and three short months later, I finally owned my very own Gold Medal Butt.

But maybe you don't care about all that. Maybe what matters most to you is how fast this program works. That the moves are simple and fun to do. That they are yours to succeed with.

You should know this: Once you decide to begin—from your very first workout—your butt has no *choice!* It cannot help but change shape. The irresistible laws of physiology are on your side. Your muscles work together. Then work against each other. Every time you flex them in each purposeful exercise, they tighten and tauten; lifting, rounding, reshaping your lower profile. They simply cannot help themselves. It's as if you'd issued them an order: "Gold Medal Butt! Take shape!"

Part of the reason results happen so fast is that our program jacks up your metabolism—and it keeps burning fat—even when you're *not* exercising. Like when you're at work or playing with the kids or even asleep. And if that's not a bonus, I don't know what is.

If you need further proof that following the program will automatically give you a Gold Medal Butt, just listen:

Not one of the fencers you see on TV, or in your town, or in the U.S. Athletic Training Center, not *one* set out to get herself a glorious bottom. She got that as a side benefit from all her parries and thrusts, her limitless lunges, and her grueling workouts. We've streamlined and simplified these movements so that they're less taxing, more fun, and more efficient.

And lucky for you, Gary's and my Gold Medal Butt Program develops in mere weeks what it took them years to accomplish.

—Mary Leonard

Our brains make us human—but our muscles make us beautiful.

I love muscles. Love them so much, I've dedicated my life to them. To the science of muscles. (That's kinesiology.) To the healing of muscles. (That's physical therapy, my lifework.) And to the training of muscles. (That's where muscles can be the most exciting, and what this book is all about.)

With Mary, my wife and cofounder of the U.S. Athletic Training Center, we heal, train, and improve the muscles of Broadway dancers, ballet stars, and college MVPs. I was the Physical Therapy Consultant to the New York Rangers hockey team for ten years and am currently affiliated with the U.S. Olympic Committee and Pro Beach Volleyball.

My practice also includes the postoperative patients of New York's greatest sports orthopedic surgeons.

Those are my credentials, but skip them. As far as you're concerned, the only thing that matters is my work with the Olympian fencers, and precisely why one noticeable part of their body is so important to you and your body.

This book will not put you "in touch with your body." (Don't you hate that smug phrase?) This book has a much more modest goal. All it will do is absolutely glorify your butt. All it will do is make you suddenly aware of six very special, very cooperative muscles that live in the neighborhood of your hips. All this book will do is take you through routines that will make your Gold Medal Butt not only possible, but inevitable. Because our Gold Medal Butt Program is not an iffy proposition. No way! These innovative exercises have been terrifically successful.

But I'm getting ahead of myself. Let's back up.

As Mary has already told you, about twelve months ago, during a training session with some Olympic athletes, she noticed something that I'd been aware of for years. Something that wouldn't surprise anyone who follows the elegant sport of fencing. Fencers, from every land, and from every race, and from every angle, have characteristically splendid butts. So if you look at a team of them, you'd have to say that while their perfect posteriors may not be rare, they certainly are exceptional.

From my schooling and experience, I knew why fencers shared this admirable feature. I'd worked for years with beginners and Gold Medal Olympians, and was painfully aware of the decades of practice, the lifetime of corrective posturing, the drill and discipline essential to this ancient sport. With all that time and training and travail, who could begrudge them their praiseworthy bottoms?

But what about people who don't fence? Who hardly had a lifetime to devote to the saber foil and epee? Why not a Gold Medal Butt for anybody, even though they'd never strut it through an Olympic village?

In short, how about you?

The answer was obvious. Because all fencers had this admirable feature, it followed that something in their training made these posterior muscles come to life and take on new shape. So, as Mary described, we figured it out and designed this program.

But the best part was perfecting these exercises, honing them, making them easier but still effective. Shortening them so they never get tedious. Making them smooth to perform, even as they work their magic. Along the way, we dropped a few that were slow to get results, and created new movements that gave us explosive rewards—dramatic and fast.

Still, this book isn't a way of life. (In fact, it's only about three months in your life.) It's not about your total body. It's single-minded, right-on-the-button, and infallibly focused on that part of your body that more people seek help for than any other. A quick solution to a longtime problem.

The program is simple, the path is true, and everything you need is enclosed within these two covers and inside your body. Your Gold Medal Butt awaits you.

Let's begin.

—Gary Guerriero

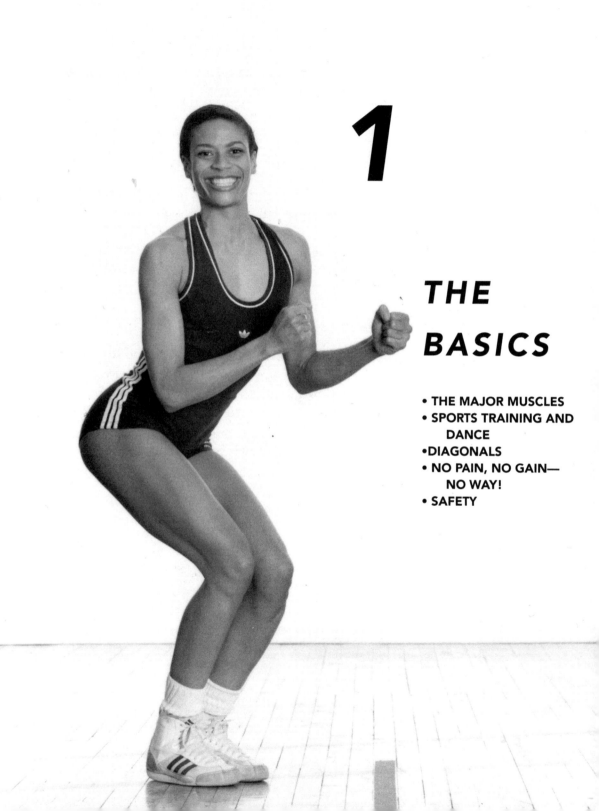

1

THE
BASICS

- THE MAJOR MUSCLES
- SPORTS TRAINING AND DANCE
- DIAGONALS
- NO PAIN, NO GAIN—NO WAY!
- SAFETY

Everything You Ever Wanted to Know About the Gold Medal Butt Program Philosophy but Were Afraid to Ask!

THE MAJOR MUSCLES YOU'RE CHANGING

Just to prove there's no mumbo-jumbo involved in this program, let's walk through a brief lesson about that crucial part of your anatomy that you are soon going to transform.

Here then are the major and important muscles you'll be working on. Note the illustrations that accompany the description so you can visualize while you exercise:

GLUTEUS MAXIMUS (opposite page)

This powerful sounding muscle is exactly that: The largest and strongest muscle you own. It contributes to your core strength, that center of gravity, balance, and action. By drawing the hip backward (acting as chief extensor), it creates the motion for walking and running. It also stabilizes the pelvis. (Otherwise you couldn't sit or get up.)

In prime condition, this beautiful muscle is gently rounded and gives subtle definition to the thigh and buttocks.

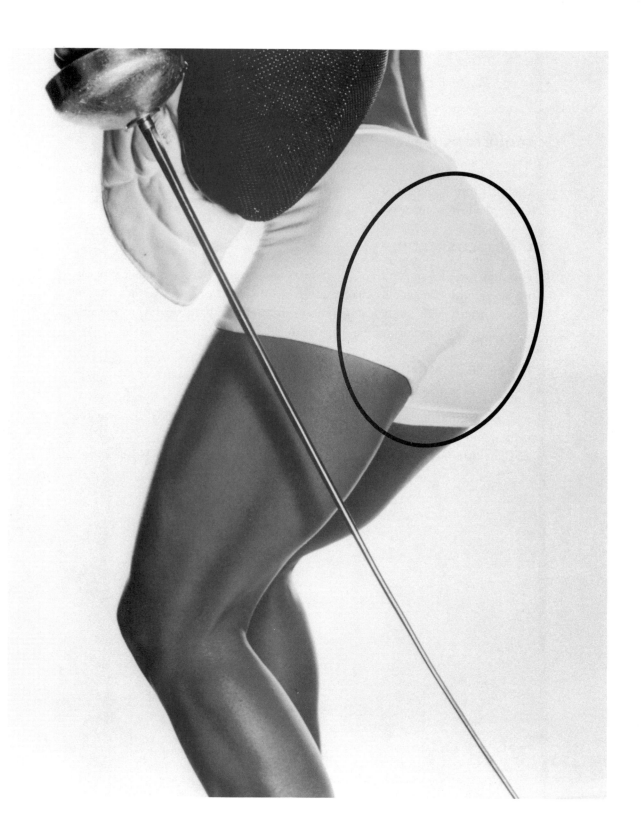

ABDUCTORS (opposite page)

Helpful, handy, and quick to improve. The abductor's biggest job is pulling the legs apart from a narrow stance. But the nicest task it performs is to add definition to the lower buttocks. The picture shows how it does its magic

1. GLUTEUS MEDIUS

This draws the leg out to the side, abducts and externally rotates the leg, working along with the gluteus maximus when you walk or run. Aesthetically, it bestows beauty with its slight indentation, imparting a light shadow to the side of the hip (and emphasizing the shape of the gluteus maximus).

2. GLUTEUS MINIMUS

This muscle is chief assistant to the medius. Although it is never seen because it is buried within the body, it must be developed because it adds shape to the medius, and grace to every motion.

These three lifelong companions are about to become your new best friends.

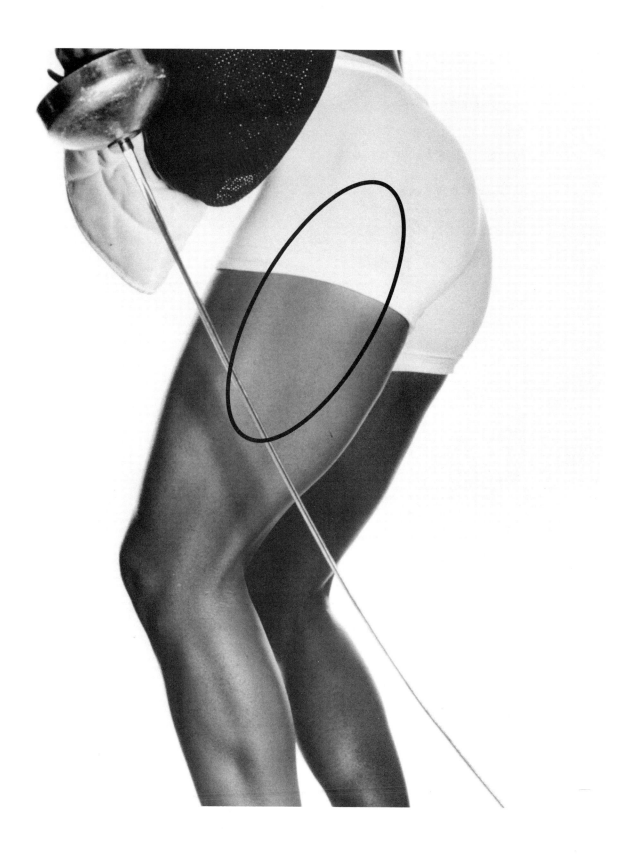

ADDUCTORS (opposite page)

These power and shape the inner thigh (they're also known as the groin muscu-lature). They break down into several muscles:

1. Adductos Longus
2. Adductos Brevis
3. Adductos Magnus
4. Gracilis

As an interactive group, they draw the thigh inward, toward the middle of the body. They also help rotate the thigh internally when turning or running.

A common injury to this group of muscles is the groin pull. That's a strain or tear caused by any violent cutting action, actually tearing the muscle fiber.

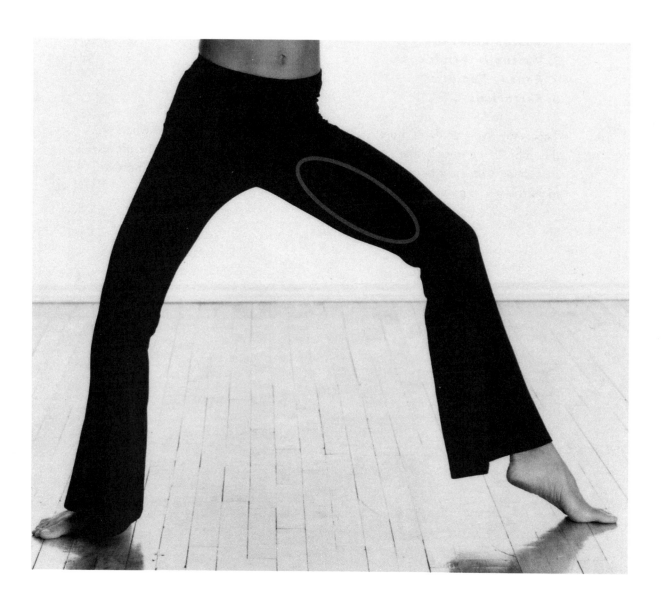

QUADRICEPS (opposite page):

1. Vastus Medialis

2. Vastus Lateralis

3. Vastus Intermidcous

4. Reutus Femoris

5. Sartorisus

This is the five-part thigh muscle, the longest muscle in your body. So what? So this: This is the muscle that's going to make it easy for you to make the moves that shape your new butt. Look at the picture, and see the dramatic improvement this guy is going to give you.

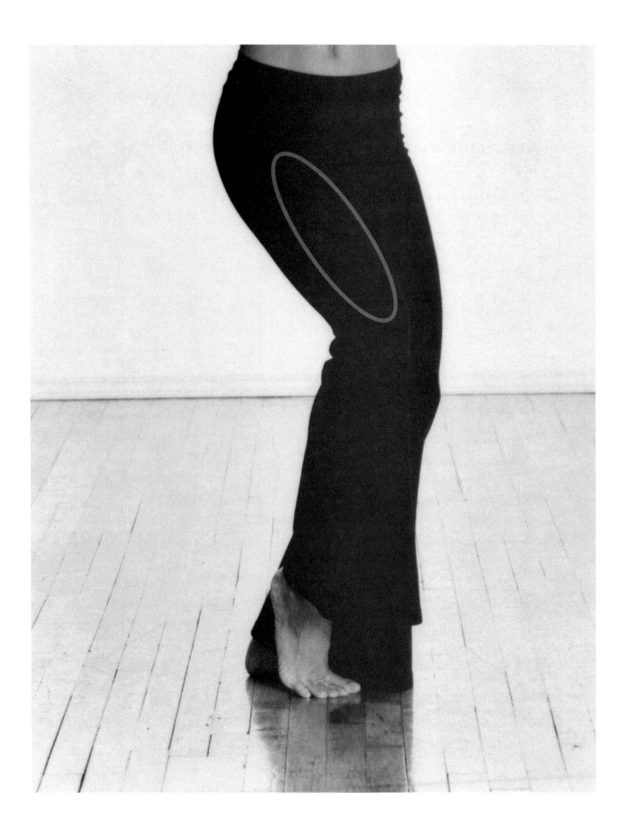

HAMSTRING MUSCLE GROUP OF POSTERIOR THIGH (opposite page)

1. Semitendonous

2. Semimembraneous

3. Biceps Femoris

All three function to extend the hip and flex the knee.

The semitendonous and semimembraneous medially rotate or internally rotate the leg.

The biceps fermoris will laterally rotate or externally rotate the leg.

All three muscles are long and chord-like in appearance, which will give you that long lean look.

A "pulled hamstring" is one of the most common muscles injured in sport.

Mechanism of injury is a violent muscular extension causing a tear or strain in the fibers of varying degrees.

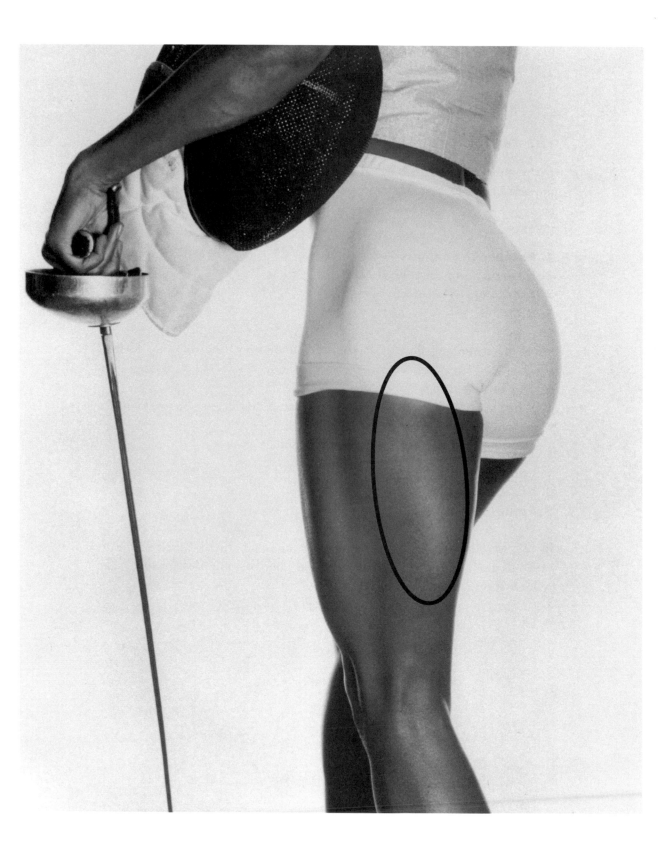

THE TRUNK (opposite page)

For purposes of your Gold Medal Butt, the trunk is what we'll call the group of muscles that control and protect your entire abdominal area and your lower back.

They are:

1. Rectus Abdominus
2. Internal and External Oblique
3. Transversus Abdominus
4. Iliopsas

All of these, working alone or in concert, function to bend the spine forward, sideways, and backward. They also stabilize the pelvis, and help the thigh musculature function properly.

When in peak condition, the well-developed abdominal region gives you that washboard stomach.

Your lower back muscles form the erector spinae group:

1. Longissiumus
2. Ilio Costilus
3. Spinalis

In addition, there is the *latissimus dorsi,* the most superficial muscle connected with this group. These defining muscles give your back the V-shape that makes your waist tiny!

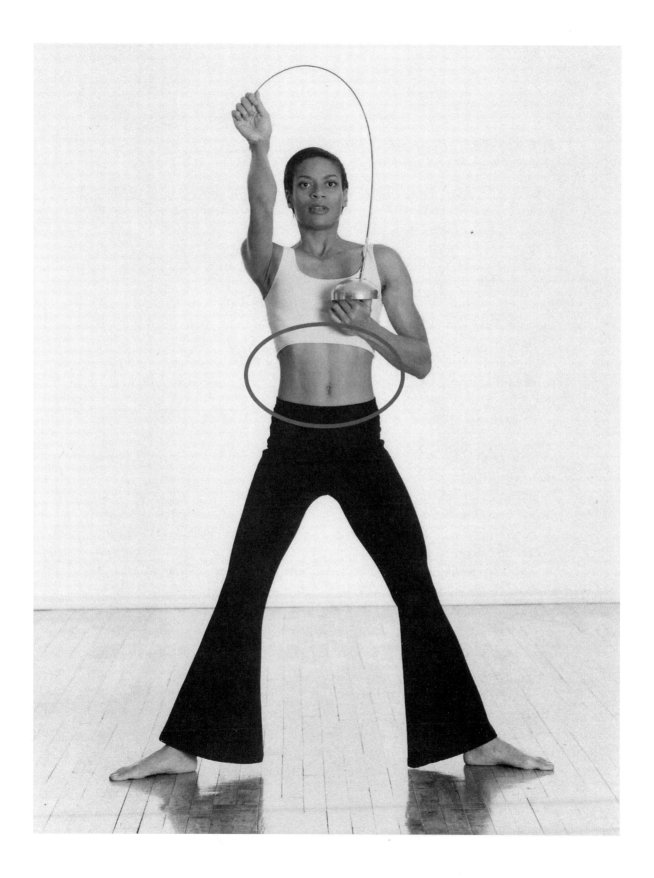

SPORTS TRAINING AND DANCE: *Not an Odd Couple, Just the Perfect Marriage!*

Mary: I grew up with four older brothers in an athletic family in Queens, New York. I learned it all—basketball, football, baseball. But I only excelled at swimming. My development as a middle-distance freestyler stopped dead the night I fell in love with Rudolf Nureyev and Margot Fonteyn.

It was June 8, 1969, and the British Royal Ballet was playing the Metropolitan Opera House in Manhattan. Nureyev and Fonteyn, the best dance team of the century, were at the height of their careers and were incredibly "on" the night I saw them in *Swan Lake.*

By their last curtain call, my fifteen-year-old life had changed. Seeing my head in a pool and swimming until my insides ached held no attraction compared to the grace, power, beauty, and raw thrills of dance. I started a life of subway rides to Manhattan for classes.

I was a theater major in college and got an M.A. in motor learning from Columbia University. Just when I thought all was well, I injured myself. I went to a lot of medical people who didn't properly address my problem. I retired early.

Blending my athletic and dance backgrounds, I was a trainer for eight years when I met Gary. Both of us having felt the pain and love of sport, my art and education and his athleticism and knowledge all seemed to blend. We've become a team that gets results.

At our gym, our clientele reflects our experience—a mixed bag of athletes, dancers, fitness novices, and weekend warriors—all striving to get in that zone where the body and mind rejoice.

We'll help you get there.

Gary: Certainly sports were the highlight of my youth, right up to college. But, slowly at first, then by leaps and bounds, my interest fastened on the science of the body, on its strengths and vulnerabilities, its limits and its vast potential. After my medical training and internship, when I began my own practice, I worked at training world-class athletes. At the same time, I was treating prima ballerinas. I discovered a strange similarity between the top athletes and the top dancers, male or female: They were all incredibly driven. And their bodies responded quickly when given the right stimuli. (How could they otherwise perform their awesome feats?) But at the same time, they all inhabited bodies that were prone to breaking down, coming up lame, pulling a hamstring, or straining a muscle. Why were they, athletes and dancers alike, so often on the injured list?

The answer, as usual, was staring me in the face: These athletes, talented to the nines and drilled to be skilled at their sport, were not trained to be *strong*. These gifted dancers, with such extraordinary control of their splendid bodies, had no real strength training in their daily regimen.

Often, the very muscle groups they needed for bursts of speed on the playing field, or for towering leaps on the stage, hadn't been strengthened to perform those tasks. They had the drive and skill to perform certain specific moves, but not the strength to withstand the strain those moves put on their body over and over again. *That* was the weakness these sports and dance athletes were hampered by. That's what made them injury prone. And that's what was shortening their careers.

And that's the secret—now the proven theory—behind the techniques Mary and I employ and teach at the U.S. Athletic Training Center. As we treat the superstars of every sport, getting them off the injured list, we do something no other training center does. Even as we cure the injury, we're also strengthening the related muscles until they're stronger than ever before.

This blending of dance finesse with the power of sports training has been utilized in your program, too. Even as you get your Gold Medal Butt, you'll feel how new strength flowing through the muscles in your center of balance makes everyday life a little smoother.

You'll be enjoying the same strengthened muscles that we give our clients. Developing enduring muscles that mean injury free years and longer careers and much more fun.

DIAGONALS

Mary: Diagonals are something I'm an absolute maniac about. I preach them and I teach them. So it should come as no surprise to you that I've slotted diagonals all through your Gold Medal Butt routines. It's no exaggeration to state that diagonals will deliver the three-dimensional roundness of the new, tight-midsectioned you. Yet most trainers never *heard* of them. Diagonals are the reason fencers look the way they do. Diagonals develop every plane of your body, and they shape your body in a way regular gym workouts can't. They add an easy completeness to each exercise. That's because they take you on a different muscular trip. Kids at play automatically use diagonals. We all did, growing up. That's what gave our young bodies their lithe angularity. Well, guess what? Diagonals will lead you right back to that lean and mean look.

All right, now instead of all this talk, let's *do* a diagonal. We'll go through simple hip isolation.

Stand up, and imagine you're standing on the middle of a face of a clock, facing 12 noon.

Now, without moving your head and shoulders, bend your knees then let your hips sway left, then right. That's hip isolation.

Next, point your right hand at 5-minutes past 12, and your left hand at 25-minutes to 12. Now let you hips move back and forth along that new line your arms are forming.

Congratulations. You have just performed your first diagonal.

That's the kind of move, done during your exercises, that will give new shape to your hips, thighs, buttocks, abs—all the major muscles we keep harping on in this program.

That's all about diagonals for now. But for the next three months, you'll be living with them.

NO PAIN, NO GAIN: The Four Words We Hate

We absolutely forbid that dangerous, reckless slogan. It is a foolish, evil lie! Listen to this, and listen good. It'll help you: Pain is not the friend of athletes or anyone else. Remember that statement because it's behind our entire training and strengthening philosophy.

We constantly teach the difference between pain and soreness and we'll teach you right now.

Soreness is the dull ache you might feel after any of the exercises in the program. The sensation lasts for a day or two at most, and it means you've activated some muscles that haven't been doing much lately. You'll feel some soreness during the first few days of your Gold Medal Butt Program, but it won't last, and truth to tell, it's kind of a satisfying feeling: It's a sign that your butt is already sitting up and starting to take notice. Soreness is a reassuring sensation that something is happening to your muscles!

Pain is different. Pain is sharp, pointed, and usually occurs when you ask too much of your body. Or when an exercise calls into play a muscle that's already injured. Not one of the exercises in your program should cause pain. So if you feel it, sharp and intensive and unmistakable, stop exercising at once. Drop back to an easier level.

And if pain persists, of course, see your doctor.

GARY ON SAFETY

Other trainers scoff at my noisy emphasis on the need for exercise that strengthens weak muscles to avoid injuries. Other trainers don't see the injuries that I treat daily; injuries caused by poor training methods.

Fact is, your body can perform incredible feats for you. And, since we strengthen as we go, your body will eventually, and easily, accomplish every exercise in the program.

That's because I very deliberately create every movement, not only to tighten and tone, but to strengthen each muscle, getting it ready for the next level. That's my tried and true way of getting you all the benefits of each workout, with little risk of injury, or even of pain.

So feel confident and enjoy each step of your program. They're designed to get you fit, and build you up for the next one, safely and surely.

Another lifelong benefit they confer is a strong lower back. (A trainload of lower back problems is almost guaranteed by some of the reckless workout videos and exercise plans on the market.)

Remember: Your body always plays fair with you. If you show it the way, it will follow. Set a challenge, and it will meet it. That's why each exercise leading to your Gold Medal Butt makes you strong enough to reach the next plateau.

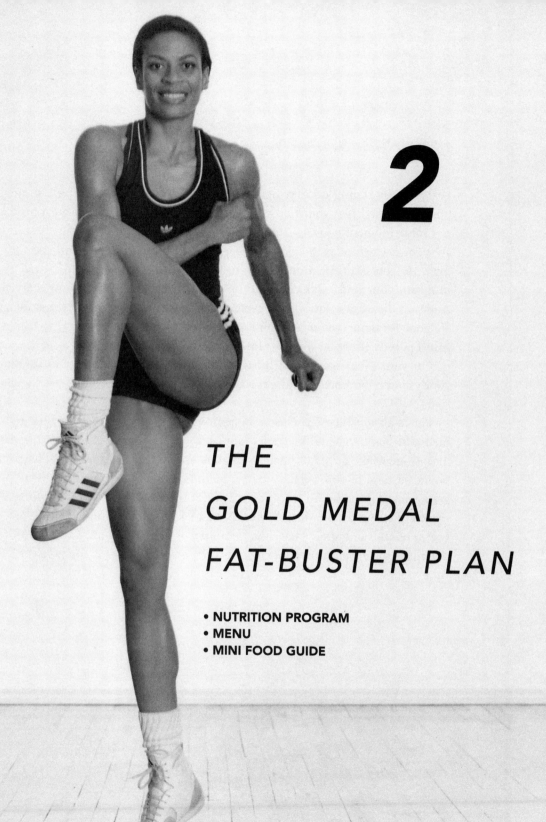

2

THE
GOLD MEDAL
FAT-BUSTER PLAN

- **NUTRITION PROGRAM**
- **MENU**
- **MINI FOOD GUIDE**

1-2-3 Fat Buster Nutrition Program

Let's start by staring calories right in the eye: Calories are nothing but energy units from food that your body uses to perform *any* activity. You burn up calories every moment you're alive, including when you're asleep. In fact, you burn away an average of 1500 calories a day, *without* exercising, if your body fat is high. As you improve your muscle-to-fat ratio during your Gold Medal Butt Program, your body will consume up to 2000 calories a day—and that's not counting the extra calories your exercises will make disappear. All those calories are gone for doing *nothing!* So on a 1500 to 2000 calories a day diet, you'd never gain a pound. (But you wouldn't lose a pound, either.)

On your Gold Medal Fat-Buster Nutrition Program, you'll also be doing your exercise movements and your aerobics. That's where results start showing, fast.

Put it all together: Fat-Buster Nutrition Program, Gold Medal Butt movement *plus* aerobics—and you're looking at a weekly calorie deficit of 3500. That means one whole *pound* of jiggling fat gone up in metabolic smoke. (That's four pounds a month, and a dandy dozen pounds lost during your ninety-day program.) Just for the fun of it, next time you're in the dairy section of your supermarket pick up a pound of butter. Now pick up four pounds. Then look at twelve pounds of butter. That's the *minimum* of what you'll lose—a whole lot of poundage that's right now blocking out the potential shape of your Gold Medal Butt.

STEP 1. Feed yourself a satisfying 20 grams of fat a day. Realistically planning, 20 grams is a lot less than you're eating now and will bust up your fat storage just fine. These days, most foods have a label listing their fat content. Read it, and correctly, by the serving. And avoid, like poison, those foods with more than 20 percent of calories from fat per serving.

HOW TO HATE EXTRA FAT

Carbohydrates and proteins pack only four calories per gram. Fat has a whopping nine calories—that's almost double!—for the same weight of food. Every time you pass up fat for the same amount of carbohydrate or protein, you get double the weight loss! Another bonus is that proteins and carbohydrates burn up 22 to 25 percent of themselves, just to be digested. Fat, on the other hand, burns only 2 to 3 percent of itself and, in addition, lards your body with the balance, since you have to either use it as energy or store it as fat.

ABOUT SUGAR

Sugar contains no fat. That's true, but sugar stops your body from *losing* fat. That's because refined sugar—candy, low-fat ice creams, pastries, etc.—release glucose into your bloodstream, forcing your body to create insulin. *That's* what inhibits the enzyme that otherwise drains fat from your fat cells. (At the same time, all that insulin makes you feel hungry. Talk about a vicious cycle!)

YOUR FAT-BUSTER 90-DAY NO-NOS

Any and all cheeses (except low-fat cottage cheese)
Fried foods
All oils
Chocolate
Mayonnaise
Sour cream
Seeds and nuts
Avocados
Beef and bacon, lamb and veal

And remember the F-sentence: *Fat falls faster if you forgo fast or fatty foods.*

STEP 2. Let's talk protein. Since you'll be building muscle to replace your fat, you need more protein than usual (the average requirement is about 50 grams a day). For a woman between 115 to 130 pounds, about 100 grams a day will do you fine. That's approximately 500 to 600 calories in protein—and will be about 40 percent of your daily caloric intake. (Obviously, the balance comes in fats and carbohydrates.)

For muscles, blood, hair, and all your internal organs to rebuild themselves, you need the eight amino acids your body itself produces and the fourteen others you get from protein. On your Fat-Buster Nutrition Program, you'll get them aplenty in egg whites, fish, and poultry, especially turkey.

Most days, you should have at least two meals with protein. If you're having fish, make sure it's low-fat, like bass, flounder, halibut, perch, or pike. Snapper, pollock, even tuna canned in water are okay. Fatty fish are out; these include catfish, herring, salmon, or mackerel. Bluefish, swordfish, and trout are not for this program. And remember: don't fry *anything*. To fill out a meal, low-fat yogurt or low-fat cottage cheese can also give you variety.

STEP 3. The complex fibrous carbohydrates are lifesavers, because you can have almost unlimited portions of broccoli, cauliflower, lettuce, green beans, eggplant, cucumber, mushrooms, squash of any variety, tomatoes, zucchini, Brussels sprouts, and spinach.

Try to cut back on starches. For the first two weeks, especially. They say that fat burns in the fire of the carbohydrate, but too much can quench the fat-flames we want to keep burning bright. So keep it down to say, one bagel or two slices of bread for the next meal, one cup of cereal or one cup of pasta, or one cup of brown rice, corn, peas, or beets. So, that's one serving at breakfast or lunch, or two at breakfast and none at lunch or dinner. Any of these satisfy your hunger, but they can put the brakes on your metabolism. So try to use them only when you're really ravenous. And absolutely no carbs at night!

Don't go hungry. If you crave a snack, give yourself a great one. Take a generous selection of those unlimited veggies listed above. Make yourself a colorful salad out of them. (Slice an apple or pear over it for an added treat.) Then sprinkle it with vinegar and freshly ground pepper, and go to town! (Daily snacks like these will also give you plenty of soluble fiber.)

And if you fall of the wagon, don't panic. A lapse is not a landslide. Just pick yourself up and start all over again.

Now that you've started your Gold Medal Butt Program, every hour, every move you make, your program is busting fat. Just burning the ugly stuff away. But that's not all. You're not just losing bulky fat, you're replacing it with sleek, shapely muscle! And that's what no program in the whole wide world can do.

Just imagine.

Let's say on a typical day, working through your program, plus your usual activity, you fat-bust 20 grams. But you eat only 10. Those other 10 grams of fat have to come from somewhere, and that means your midsection and other places. Ten grams of fat gone forever!

And that equation works like a charm, unstoppably, every day for the next three months. You'll take in less fat than you burn up, and your body must grab the flab from yourself—hateful flab that's the only thing between you and your Gold Medal Butt.

Now copy this next paragraph and stick it on your refrigerator, on your breadbox, on your pillow, even *memorize* it. Because it is a breathtaking concept: Follow your Fat-Buster feedings. Follow your exercise for a half-hour at a time. And every three weeks, you'll be four or five pounds lighter. And as all that fat gets busted away, you'll keep getting sleeker, more contoured, more Gold Medal Butt-like.

Finally, let's talk about vitamins and minerals. Natural or supplements? We all get our vitamins from food, and our minerals from food and inorganic compounds. Many studies support the belief that a diet rich in complex carbohydrates, fresh fruits, and low-fat protein supplies all the vitamins and minerals you need. Other health experts swear by supplements. And a visit to any health food store will show you that the supplement message is being heard and heeded by many.

For the purposes of your Gold Medal Butt Program, here's a simple rule: If you're not sure whether you want to take supplements, show this plan to your doctor or trainer—or call us. (Always a good idea before *any* new exercise program.) Then the two of you can decide which supplements you may want to add to your diet.

YOUR FAT-BUSTING MENU

The Ten Fat-Busting Starters for Your Program

These meals are surprisingly satisfying, and they'll give you plenty of energy and stamina. Each one breaks down into approximately 40 percent protein, 40 percent carbohydrate, and 20 percent fat. As the weeks go on, you can substitute one meal for the other, even go outside the diet to other vegetables and fruits as you prefer. Mix and match and use this menu as a blueprint for the three-month program—and beyond!

A Fat-Busting Secret

Try to eat dinner no later than 6 P.M. This keeps your body busting fat for several hours before bedtime and speeds your metabolism up, making fat fall away even faster. (No carbs after 6 P.M.)

The Best Way to Lose Water? Drink Lots of Water!

Sounds crazy, but it's true. Drinking lots of water flushes the sodium out of your system. Sodium makes you retain water, so when it's gone, lots of water is released right along with it. Drink eight to twelve 8-ounce glasses of real, pure water every day. Don't count coffee, tea, soft drinks, or soup. Good water also curbs your appetite. (Hunger is sometimes thirst in disguise. Drink a glass of water and sometimes hunger disappears.) If all this isn't good enough for you, water also clears up your complexion. Take a good close look about three days after you begin drinking your eight to twelve glasses. You'll be very nicely surprised.

The Two Fibers: Friends Indeed!

On your Fat-Buster Nutrition Program, you'll get both kinds of fiber:

Soluble Fiber

This comes from fruit, vegetables, legumes, and psyllium. These fibers lower body sugar, lower cholesterol levels, and even carry cholesterol with them when they leave your body.

Insoluble Fiber

You get this from whole wheat and grains, corn, brown rice, potato skin, and green leafy vegetables. You can't digest it, but it bulks up your stool and helps prevent constipation. Even better, it actually helps rid your body of fat. That's because as it moves through your digestive track, it transports excess fat along with it. And good riddance!

Cellulite: Ugh!

It's common, it's dimpled, it's a form of fat, and it's as unattractive as flesh can get. Lots of people think this spongy stuff is permanent. Well, it's not. You're going to see your cellulite disappear from your thighs and midsection as you start achieving your Gold Medal Butt. That's because all your exercises and your aerobics create muscles in the places now occupied by cellulite. Every movement you make helps burn away the cellulite fat wherever it's hitching a ride on your body. Cellulite *can* be met and conquered and you're going to prove it.

A Word to Anyone Out There Who Is Heavy

The Gold Medal Butt Program won't make you skinny, but listen to this: You'll be surprised at how many of the movements you can perform at first, how many more you'll be able to perform as the days zip by, how good all this activity is going to make you feel—and how much your appetite will drop.

On the Fat-Buster Nutrition Program, you'll lose a lot more than some others, because you've got more to lose. But your increased strength, your improved circulation, your stirred muscles are going to give you a determination you've never before had. It's happened before. This time let it happen to *you*!

YOUR FAT-BUSTING MENU

DAY ONE **BREAKFAST**

> 2 egg white omelet, with basil and chopped tomato
> 2 slices whole wheat toast
> 8 oz. fruit juice, or a whole apple or pear

LUNCH

> 6-8 oz. grilled chicken breast (A *big* hint: Cut cooked chicken breast
> into chunks and wrap each in a leaf of lettuce. It tastes great, adds no
> calories, and really stretches that chicken.)
> 2 cups steamed or fresh broccoli or squash (or *both)*
>
> An orange, apple, or pear and any herbal tea

SNACK

> 1 cup of low-fat yogurt

DINNER

> 6-8 oz. grilled fresh tuna
> 1 cup cooked spinach (or any other favorite vegetable)
> 1 piece of fruit
> Mineral water

DAY TWO **BREAKFAST**

> 1 cup of cereal with 8 oz. skim milk
> 1 slice of whole wheat toast
> 8 oz. fruit juice

LUNCH

1 cup low-fat cottage cheese
½ head of any type of lettuce
2 cups fresh fruit salad

Fat-Buster Hint: Use that lettuce as a bed, first for the cottage cheese, then for the fruit salad—it makes the meal much more satisfying.

SNACK

1 oz. pretzels with mineral water. Of course you can drink mineral water all day. Up to eight 8-oz. glasses.

DINNER

One 4-8 oz. broiled or grilled flounder filet
½ cup carrots,
½ cup spinach or squash
Dessert: 1 cup blueberries. One at a time. Make them last.

DAY THREE BREAKFAST

Coffee or tea
8 oz. fruit juice
½ cup cooked cereal. Add sliced banana, cinnamon, or nutmeg
1 slice of whole wheat toast

LUNCH

4-6 oz. turkey, cut into squares, each wrapped in a lettuce leaf
1 cup pasta
½ melon
Mineral water or herbal tea

SNACK

1 grapefruit, sprinkled with cinnamon and broiled. Delicious.

DINNER

3 oz. broiled or grilled tile fish
12 Brussels sprouts
½ cup turnips
1 piece of fruit

DAY FOUR **BREAKFAST**

3 egg white omelet. Add pepper and 1 tsp. mustard for color and zest.
1 slice whole wheat toast
1 cup nonfat milk.

LUNCH

1½ cups sliced fruit
½ cup plain yogurt or low-fat cottage cheese
2 rice cakes
Herbal tea

SNACK

1 cup nonfat milk with ½ cup orange juice. (With 4 ice cubes in a blender and you've got a great drink!)

DINNER

4 oz. grilled lean ground steak patty, on 1 slice whole wheat toast
3 cups salad, with ½ tsp. olive oil and balsamic vinegar
Apple, pear, or orange sections for dessert

DAY FIVE **BREAKFAST**

Yogurt shake: Combine 1 cup nonfat yogurt, ¾ cup chopped melon, 4 ice cubes, and ½ cup juice of choice in a blender—a great breakfast!
Herbal tea

LUNCH

½ cup pasta
1 cup tomato sauce
Grilled or steamed vegetables, all you want from the list—add to pasta and sauce for huge bowl of *lunch*!
Mineral water
Herbal tea

DINNER

4-6 oz. white meat turkey, with sprinkles of lemon or vinegar
Large lettuce and tomato salad
Sliced pear, heated with cinnamon

DAY SIX **BREAKFAST**

3 egg white omelet, with ½ tsp. mustard, on 1 slice of whole wheat toast
½ tsp. no-sugar-added jam on a slice of toast for a treat
8 oz. fresh juice

LUNCH

Large salad, 2 or 3 cups, with lemon, vinegar, and dry mustard dressing
4-6 oz. white tuna packed in water. Sprinkle half on top of salad, half on 1 slice of toast
Herbal tea

SNACK

Sliced apple and orange salad

DINNER

4-6 oz. grilled chicken
1 cup of steamed mixed vegetables: broccoli, carrots, celery, green beans
Fruit shake: Add 6 strawberries and ½ banana with 1 cup of water and
4 ice cubes to the blender and mix

DAY SEVEN **BREAKFAST**

1 cup of blueberries, or any favorite berries
3 pancakes made with skim milk, sprinkled with cinnamon or nutmeg
Herbal tea or coffee

LUNCH

4-6 oz. grilled, skinned chicken, chopped in chunks, and wrapped in
lettuce with steamed broccoli florets
2 cups tomato and onion salad, with ½ tsp. oil and vinegar dressing
Herbal tea

SNACK

½ yogurt shake (see Day 5)

DINNER
Fresh fruit salad
1 cup carrot or vegetable soup
1 cup nonfat yogurt, mixed with diced apple
Herbal tea

DAY EIGHT **BREAKFAST**

3 egg white omelet, with ½ tsp. mustard, 1 small potato, and mushrooms
1 slice whole wheat toast

1 cup of juice
Herbal tea

LUNCH

5 oz. broiled or poached filet of sole, with lemon slices
Fresh green salad
1 melon of choice
Herbal tea

SNACK

15 mushrooms, sliced, and sautéed in 2 tbs. water, drained and served on 1 slice of whole wheat toast with a dash of Dijon mustard. *Tasty!*

DINNER

4 oz. lean meatloaf on a bed of lettuce, sliced tomato, and diced onion
1 cup steamed or boiled broccoli
½ cup steamed carrots
1 sliced orange, sprinkled with cinnamon
Herbal tea

DAY NINE **BREAKFAST**

1 cup oatmeal, with ¼ cup raisins and ½ cup warm skim milk
8 oz. orange juice
Herbal tea or coffee

LUNCH

1 cup pasta, with 3 oz. grilled chicken with vegetables
½ melon of choice
Herbal tea or coffee

SNACK

Chopped apple with a sprinkle of walnuts, about 1 tsp. Delish!

DINNER

4-6 oz. white meat turkey, in chunks, mixed with 1 tbs. fresh cran-
berries, and wrapped in lettuce leaves
½ acorn squash, with 2 tbs. fresh dill
1½ cups fresh fruit
Herbal tea or coffee

DAY TEN **BREAKFAST**

Big Shake: In a blender, combine 8 oz. orange juice, 1 cup sliced
pineapple, 1 cup strawberries, ½ banana. Add 5 ice cubes and blend
away!
2 slices whole wheat toast
Herbal tea or coffee.

LUNCH

3 cups salad, plus 4 hard-boiled egg whites, dressed with lots of pepper,
½ tsp. olive oil, and 1 tbs. balsamic vinegar
½ melon of choice

SNACK

1 diced pear tossed with ½ cup nonfat yogurt

DINNER

4-6 oz. grilled monkfish
2 cups steamed vegetables of choice
Herbal tea

Below you'll find a food guide chart that will give you a sense of what is in some of the foods we're recommending. For a more complete guide, we suggest you pick up one of the many calorie-counter books available at your supermarket or bookstore.

Enjoy!

FOOD	CALORIES	PROTEIN	FAT	CARBS
1 slice of wheat bread	70	3	1	12
1 egg white	17	3.5	0	0.3
8 oz. orange juice	100	1.3	0.4	19.3
Herbal tea	2	0	0	1
Coffee	4	0.1	0	0.8
Canned, light tuna in water	90	12	1	0
4 oz. fresh tuna	158	34	1.4	0
2 cups boiled spinach	42	5.4	0.4	6.8
1 apple	81	6	0.5	21.1
4 oz. light meat chicken	196	35.1	5.1	0
2 cups broccoli	88	9.2	0.8	15.6
1 cup low-fat yogurt	190	8	6	36
½ melon	84	2.1	0.6	19.6
8 oz. apple juice	110	1.3	0.4	19
1 cup pasta	240	10.7	0.9	39

FOOD	CALORIES	PROTEIN	FAT	CARBS
1 cup tomato sauce	74	3.2	0.8	16.8
1 cup carrots	70	1.8	1	16.2
4 oz. turkey	93	66.4	11.2	0
½ head any type of lettuce	35	2.7	0.5	5.7
1 pear	98	0.7	0.7	25.1
1 cup oatmeal	145	6	2.4	25.2
1 cup skim milk	86	8.4	0.4	11.9
1 cup low-fat cottage cheese	200	28	4	8
1 oz. pretzels	108	2.6	1	22.5
4 oz. flounder	104	21.4	1.4	0
1 cup Brussels sprouts	60	4	0.8	13.6
1 cup mashed turnips	42	1.6	0.2	11.2
½ grapefruit	37	0.7	0.1	8.2
1 rice cake	50	1	3	12

FOOD	CALORIES	PROTEIN	FAT	CARBS
¼ lean hamburger	217	32	8.3	0
½ cup chopped tomato	19	0.8	0.3	4.2
¼ cup raisins	125	1.5	0	33

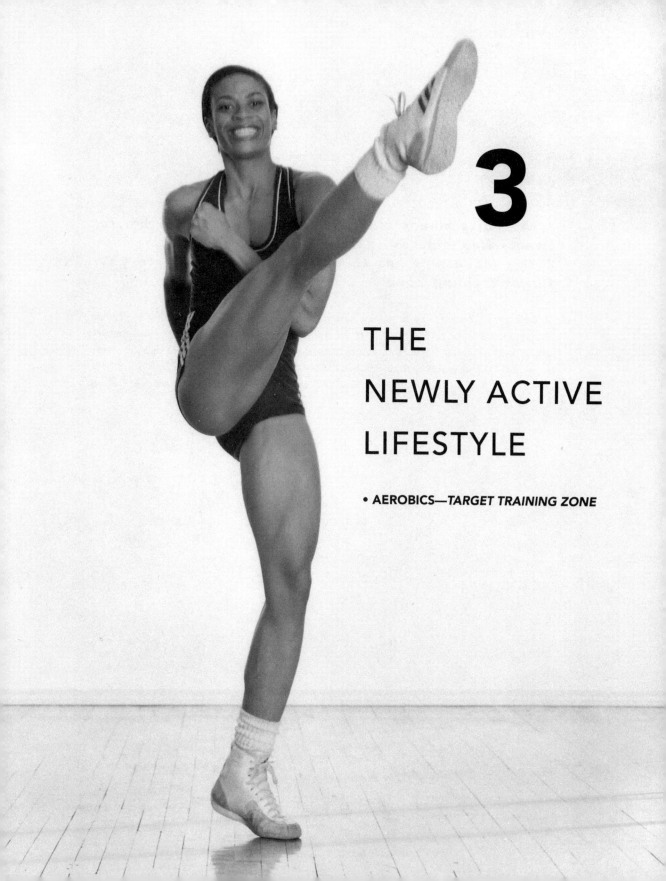

3

THE
NEWLY ACTIVE
LIFESTYLE

• AEROBICS—TARGET TRAINING ZONE

AEROBICS

1. Aerobics means moving in some chosen rhythm for twenty-five minutes or more.
2. This movement has to push your pulse rate to your Target Training Zone.

To calculate your Target Training Zone, subtract your age from 220. Then, find 70 percent of that number. Now, find 90 percent of the number. The range between these two numbers is your Target Training Zone. Your aerobics should push your pulse to a rate between these two numbers. *(For example, for a thirty-six-year-old the formula would be: 220 - 36 = 184; 184 x .7 = 128.8; 184 x .85 = 156.4. Therefore, the Target Training Zone would be 128.8–156.4.)*

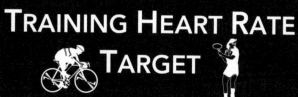

TRAINING HEART RATE TARGET

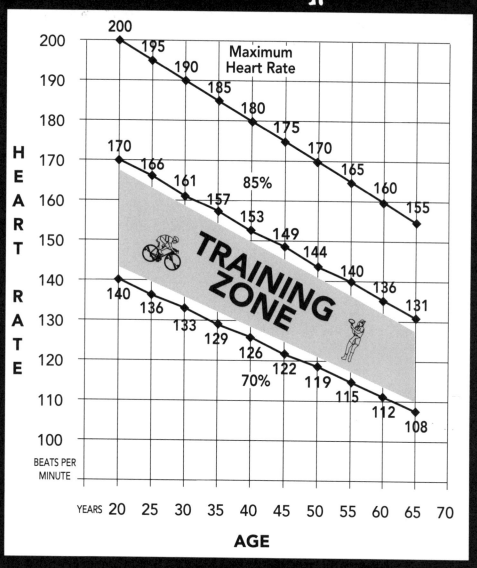

Maximum
Heart Rate

200
195
190
185
180
175
170
166
165
161
160
157
155
153
149
144
140
136
131

170
140
136
133
129
126
122
119
115
112
108

85%

70%

TRAINING ZONE

HEART RATE

200
190
180
170
160
150
140
130
120
110
100

BEATS PER
MINUTE

YEARS 20 25 30 35 40 45 50 55 60 65 70

AGE

The information contained in this chart is based on guidelines set forth by the American Heart Association.

The reason we add aerobics to your Gold Medal Butt Program is that these steady, no-rest, twenty-five-minute chunks of activity improve the health of your heart and lungs. At the same time, aerobics burns away still more of your unwanted fat.

The aerobics you choose to perform should repeat the body rhythms of the activities you like best: walking, jogging, skating, swimming, fast dancing, biking, jumping rope, hiking, cross-country skiing, or rowing. Or vary them.

It doesn't matter what you do, as long as it gets your heartbeat up to your Target Training Zone, and you keep at it for twenty-five minutes or more. (Continue it for thirty-five minutes or more, and you'll just burn away that much more fat, replacing it with sleek, slenderizing muscle. Ideally, if you have the time and energy, go for one hour.) One beautiful, healthful side of aerobics is how soon you become conditioned to performing them without stopping for a rest. Even if you puff a little the first day or two, your shortness of breath will soon disappear. Instead, your body will switch to the deep, rhythmic breathing that challenges your lungs and heart. *And* these aerobics make your Gold Medal exercises easier to perform.

Do your aerobics three times a week on the days you're not working out (or, if you have the time, just do it right after exercising). It's a half-hour that you'll treasure!

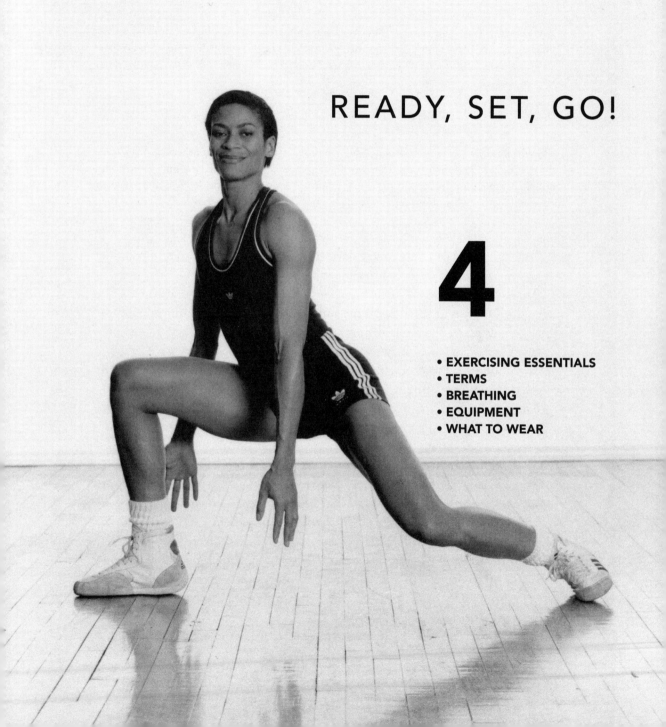

READY, SET, GO!

4

- **EXERCISING ESSENTIALS**
- **TERMS**
- **BREATHING**
- **EQUIPMENT**
- **WHAT TO WEAR**

How to Get Extra Shapeliness with No Extra Work!

This is easy, and it really pays off. When you do an exercise in the program, feel, or isolate, which of the six major muscles you're moving. Once you feel it, concentrate on it, notice how it's performing. This simple trick of paying attention to each muscle will make each workout twice as effective. You're welcome.

Why Nothing Beats the Beauty of the Butt

A Gold Medal Butt lends proportion to your profile. It adds grace to your stride and balance to your stature. Because it is buttressed with complex layers of muscle, any butt can develop striking contours. And since it is the only part of the body that can be deliberately shaped by these exercises, it will go from formless and jiggly to alluring and curvaceous.

Here is your complete Gold Medal Butt Home Exercise Program.

Your program takes only ninety days, but you perform these exercises on only thirty-six days out of the entire three months!

Three times a week. That's all it takes. On three alternate days (or on the same day each week) you'll perform your aerobics. So set those three half-hour time periods aside. Then guard those thirty-minute segments like a tigress protects her cubs. For the next twelve weeks those periods belong to *you*. (If you've got a faithful friend to do the program with you, so much the better. You'll correct and inspire each other.)

The number of sets and reps for all these exercises stay the same for the entire first month. Even though each exercise will grow easier as the days swiftly pass, you should concentrate on *concentrating*. Focus on isolating the muscle you're working on. Feel it on your body, and see it in your mind.

Improve your performance of each movement. Take the time to release more *slowly*. Perfect the smoothness of your breathing. Finally, gradually decrease your rest periods between each set. And fill any time left over in your half-hour—or spice up your routine—with extra exercises from the Gold Medal Optionals.

Also, take a look ahead at the Special Trunk and Abdominal Strengthening and Stretches chapters to round out your program. A tighter stomach will enhance your butt. And stretching keeps the body limber and feels *very good* after a good workout.

After all this talk, the moment of truth has arrived. You are embarking on a grand and glorious journey that will take only three months, but, oh, the changes in store! Your Gold Medal Butt Program is broken down into three segments, each one preparing you for the next one.

Then there's the fourth part, a gym-based program preparing you for a lifetime of you looking and feeling better, clothes fitting better, and your every move showing a new awareness of your core, your center, your point of balance.

You'll notice. Your friends will notice. The whole world will notice.

EXERCISING ESSENTIALS

TERMS

1: **Isolation** of a muscle. This simply means making you focus on a specific muscle. So you can feel it relax when you release it. Isolation means you can concentrate on that single muscle as you work it and feel it develop.

2: **Flexing** a muscle. This means putting a muscle to work. As you make a muscle, you are "flexing" a bicep. As you squeeze your buttocks together, you are developing tension in or contracting the gluteus maximus. Simple enough, eh?

3: **Release**. This means relaxing the muscle or muscles you've just flexed. In every case, when we say "release," relax that muscle *slowly*. Don't just let it drop. And as you'll see, every little bit helps.

4: A **Repetition** or **Rep**. This is the performance of a single exercise. Stand up on your toes right now, hold 2 counts, and come back down. You just did a rep.

5: A **Set**. This is a given number of reps for any exercise. Stand up on your toes and come down right now, three times in a row. You just did a set with three reps. See how good you're getting already?

6: **Prone** and **Supine**. Prone just means lying face down. Supine means lying face up. You'll be doing both.

7: **The Readiness Position.** Your very best friend—this is a relaxed and balanced stance. Your feet are slightly more than shoulder width apart, your face and eyes looking straight ahead, your knees not locked, hands at your side. Your whole posture is ready for anything. Give yourself a nice shake, and see how good it feels.

BREATHING

It seems as if it would be the simplest of life's tasks, and impossible to do improperly. Seems like. Actually, as we'll stress many times in this book, proper breathing is both necessary and *helpful* in performing all the movements.
Other rules are simple, but strict:

1. Avoid apical, or top-of-the-chest, breathing.
2. Always isolate the abdominal muscles as you breathe.

Here's a simple exercise that shows exactly the technique of breathing you should strive for:
1: Lie on your bed or on the floor. Put both your hands over your lower abdomen. Push your hands down as you slowly breathe out, slowly pulling your belly button toward your spine. (But *not* throwing your chest out. just push your stomach flat.) Now inhale slowly, steadily, but not letting your chest inflate. Instead, relax your abdominals so a Santa Claus–like belly grows under your hands.

That's the kind of deep breathing you'll want to do through your routine. It gives you lots of oxygen, and also expels stale air from your lungs. Also, try to get the hang of inhaling through the nose and exhaling through the mouth. (At first, you may not seem to be getting enough air in, but it will soon be comfortable and natural.) Breathing this way will also prevent hyperventilation, which is too much oxygen in the blood and can result in dizziness and fainting.

One final thing to keep in mind about breathing: Always *inhale* as you set yourself for the exercise. Always *exhale* as you exert yourself in the exercise.

EQUIPMENT

The complete, total, comprehensive list of home equipment you'll need to achieve your Gold Medal Butt:

1. A bath towel
2. A kitchen chair
3. A small pillow

The only equipment you'll have to buy:

1. A set of ankle weights, preferably with Velcro fasteners, that are adjustable to 20 pounds.
2. A set of adjustable dumbbells, total weight 30 pounds.

WHAT TO WEAR?

Sneakers, sweats or leotards, walking shoes, T-shirt, whatever makes you nice and comfortable as you work out and that you can toss in the wash afterward. A headband can help in some of the positions.

So put on your workout duds, turn up some music, and clear a space in your room.

The time has come.

Let's begin!

STRETCHING

After exercising, be sure to stretch that body (see Chapter 11)!

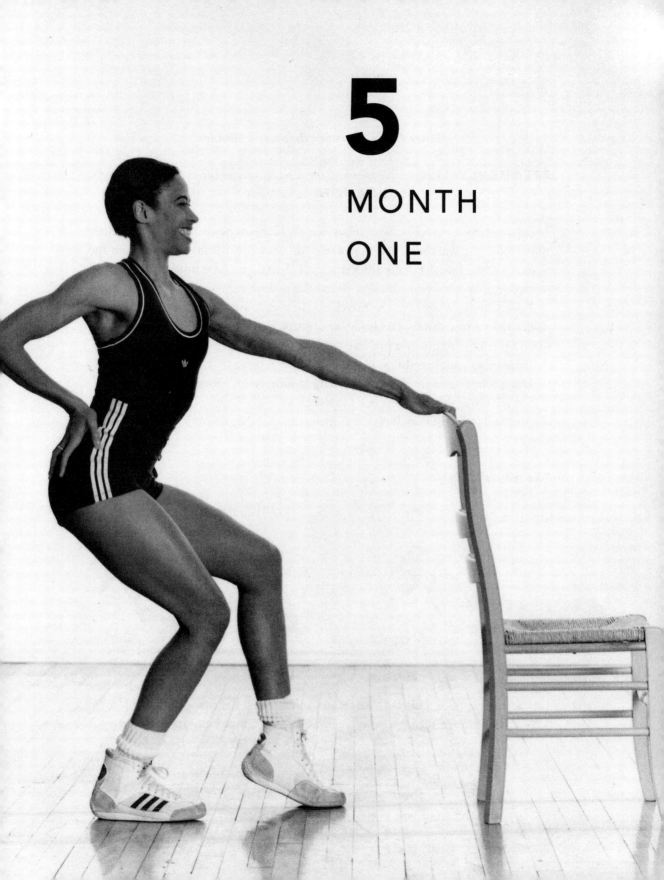

5

MONTH
ONE

Where Every Beginner Becomes a Winner!

FREQUENCY: Monday, Wednesday, and Friday (or any three alternating days).
DURATION: 30 minutes.

There are twelve exercises here. They are all to be done in the thirty minutes allotted for the workout. The first week you may not be able to complete the routine. That's fine. Just take the extra time. Soon, you'll be finishing more and more, until, by week two, you'll be doing the daily dozen.

Rest thirty seconds between exercises. (In every case, if you feel up to it, just jangle your arms, shake your body, and move right into the next exercise. It'll speed up your workout and increase the aerobic effect.)

Remember your breathing. Inhale as you get set; exhale as you exert.

Don't forget your abs and trunk strengthening (see Chapter 10).

Stretch after your workout (see Chapter 11).

And maintain your cardiovascular program!

The Elvis-Pelvis

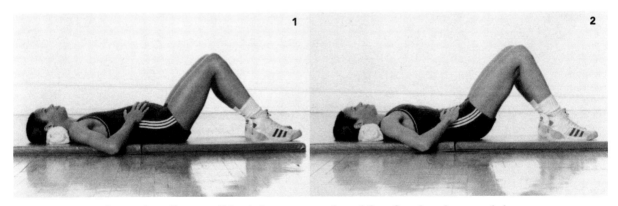

Lie face up on floor. Pull both knees up, soles of feet flat, hands over abdomen. Take a deep breath through your nose, and feel a Santa Belly form under your hands (see Position **1**). Now let your muscles push your belly-button toward your spine. At the same time, squeeze buttocks, tilt pelvis toward ceiling (see Position **2**). Hold for 2 seconds. (Say "One Guerriero, two Guerriero.") Now release your buttocks, *slowly,* along with your entire body. You just did the pelvic tilt, a move that recurs a lot in this program and works full-time wonders.

Now repeat that same movement 4 more times, or reps. Rest 10 seconds.

Do 3 more sets of 5 reps each.

LEG RAISES

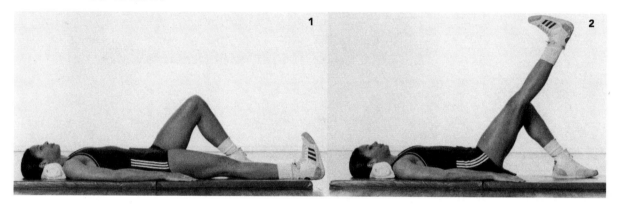

Lie face up, left leg bent at the knee, with the sole of foot flat on the floor (see Position **1**). Extend right leg, foot flexed, with toes pointed toward head, and lift leg to height of left knee (see Position **2**). Hold for 2 seconds. *Slowly* release. Perform 7 more reps. Then 4 sets of 8 reps each.

Repeat same exercise for left leg.

Checkpoint for Leg Raises

Keep lower back pressed to the floor throughout by pressing belly button to spine. Do *not* hyperextend (bow upward) either leg.

SIDE-LYING ADDUCTION

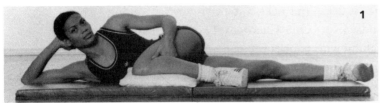

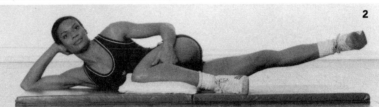

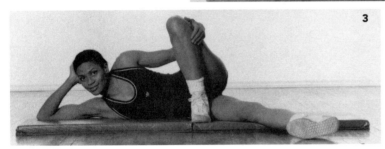

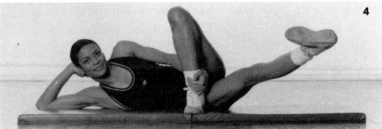

Lie on your right side, head in hand, left knee pulled up toward chest. Place pillow under left knee. (This protects your lower back.) Now place left hand under left knee, pull belly button toward spine. It's easy (see Position **1**).

Flex right toe toward head, keeping foot facing forward throughout movement. Lock right knee, breathe properly, and raise right leg as high as possible, 8 inches or more (see Position **2**). Hold for 2 seconds. Release *slowly.* Do 7 more reps.

Then lie on right side, head in hand, left knee to chest, pillow under left knee, left hand under left knee. Repeat exercise, doing 4 sets of 8 reps each, alternating sides.

Checkpoint for Side-lying Adduction

Keep foot pointed straight out.

Your first Diagonal! (Reread page **16** to refresh your memory.) Lie on your right side. Put your right leg at the 4 o'clock position. Fold left leg over left and secure with left hand (see Position **3**). Lift right leg 8 inches or higher (see Position **4**). Hold for a 2 count. Slowly release.

Alternate right and left sides, doing 4 sets of 8 reps each. These diagonals really emphasize that contouring. Can't you feel it?

SIDE-LYING ABDUCTION

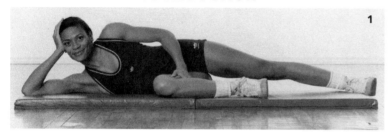

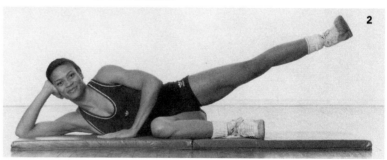

Lie on right side, head in right hand. Right leg pulled to chest, with left hand on floor (see Position **1**). Lift right leg, flexed, 6–12 inches (see Position **2**). Hold for a 2 count. Slowly release. Repeat 8 times. Repeat for left side. Do 4 sets, 8 reps each, alternating sides.

Checkpoint for Side-lying Abduction

Keep moving leg flexed, and note how foot is pointed straight out.

HIP EXTENSION

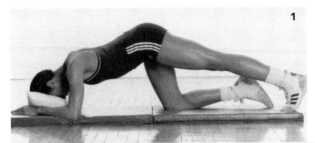

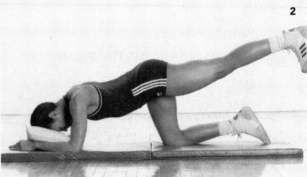

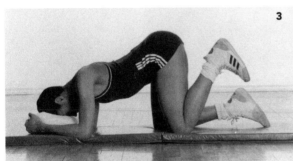

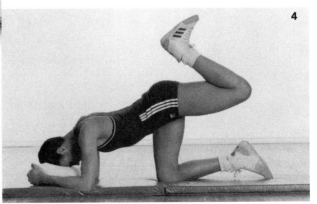

Support yourself on your knees and elbows, hands flat on floor, head resting on a pillow (see Position **1**). Flex right foot, raise leg in line with body, approaching a 45-degree angle (see Position **2**). Hold for 2 seconds. *Slowly* release. Do 4 sets of 5 reps for both right and left legs. (This is fabulous for the buttocks and works wonders for the posterior thighs.)

Adopt the same position as above, but this time, flex your right foot, getting heel as close as possible to buttock (see Position **3**). Raise your right leg by contracting or squeezing *right* buttock, till right thigh is parallel to floor (see Position **4**).

Hold for 2 seconds. Release. Do 4 sets of 8 reps each, alternating legs.

Checkpoint for Hip Extension

Remember to keep your belly button pressed to your spine. Don't let your body get out of line.

LEG PRESS

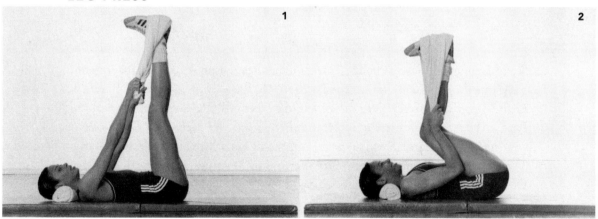

Use two towels. Roll one up and place it behind your neck for comfort and support. Place the other towel across heels and grip with both hands, legs extended (see Position **1**). Now bend knees to chest (see Position **2**). Now, pushing by squeezing buttocks, *not* thighs, push back to Position **1**. Using the buttocks instead of the thighs works much better for your butt. Do 4 sets of 8 reps each.

STANDING HIP EXTENSION AT CHAIR

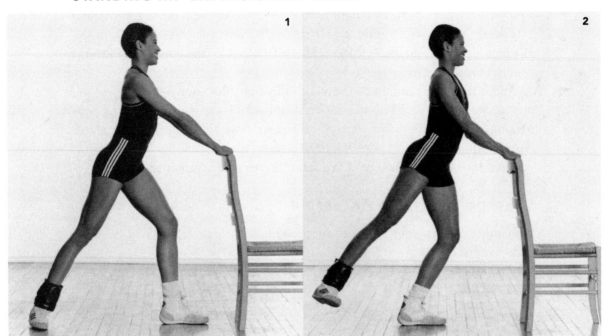

Stand facing the back of the chair, with hands resting on its back. Face forward, belly button pressed to spine (see Position **1**). Raise your right foot, flexed, 12 inches from floor (see Position **2**). Hold 2 seconds. Release. Repeat 8 times. Repeat the exercise for left foot. Do 4 sets of 8 reps for each leg. (The model is wearing ankle weights, which we recommend only when this becomes easy. Then use 1-pound ankle weights and increase by 1 pound every fourth workout. Don't worry, next month you'll be using ankle weights a lot more!)

Checkpoint for Standing Hip Extension

To ensure your body is in proper alignment, stand so you *could* raise yourself on the ball of your supporting foot at any time. This will help you keep your body from drifting right or left.

STANDING LEG CURL

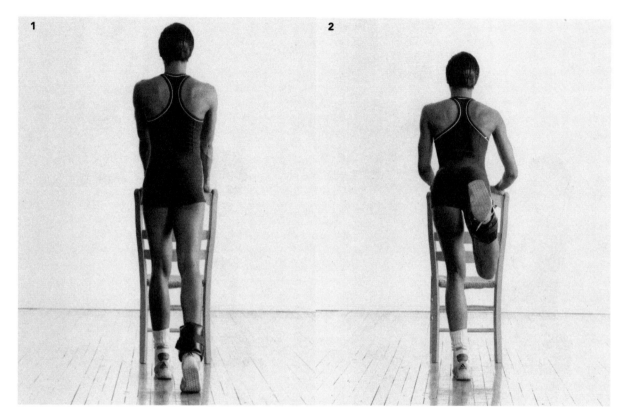

Stand facing the back of the chair, with hands resting on its back. Left knee slightly bent, right toe on floor (see Position **1**). Keep your right foot flexed, and raise heel as close as possible to your contracted buttocks (see Position **2**). Hold for 2 seconds. Slowly return. Do 4 sets of 8 reps each, for each leg.

Checkpoint for Leg Curl

Do *not* stick out your buttocks on this movement. *Do not bend forward!* If you do, the exercise will be of almost no value.

CALF RAISE

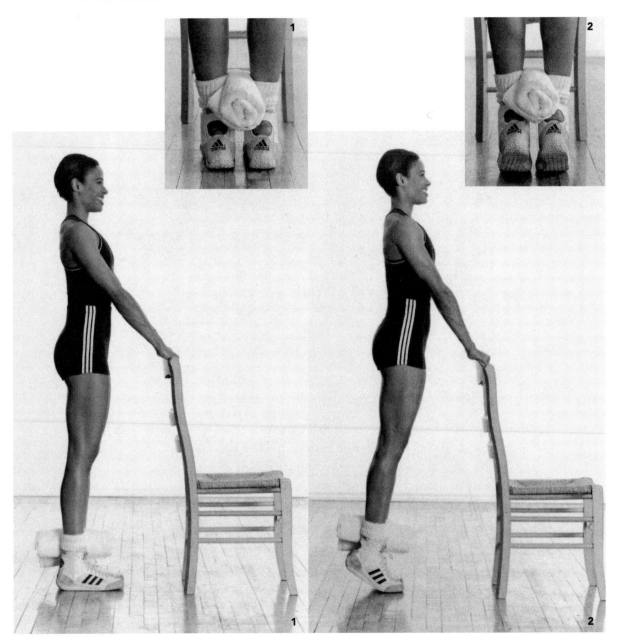

Place a rolled up towel between your ankles (see Close-ups **1** and **2**). This maintains proper foot alignment and prevents strain on ankle joint. Assume the readiness position. Belly button to spine (see Position **1**). Squeeze your buttocks tight as you rise up on the balls of your feet (see Position **2**). Use the chair for balance, but *not* for support. Hold for a 2 count, then lower yourself. Keep buttocks and all other muscles you can feel down the back of the legs contracted as you lower yourself to the floor.

Checkpoint for Calf Raise

As you rise to the ball of your foot, keep your weight on your big toe and the one next to it. And keep that towel clenched between your ankles. That stops your feet from rolling out.

CHAIR JAZZ SQUAT

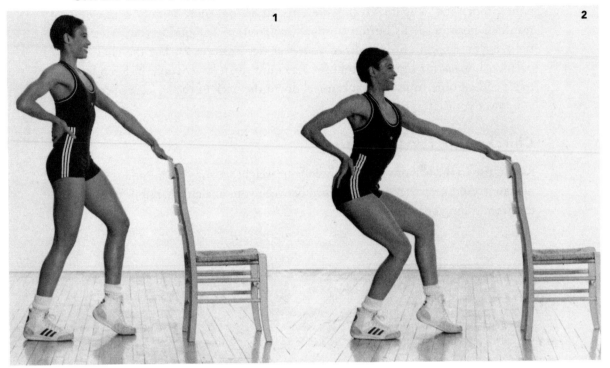

This is a diagonal.

Stand facing the back of the chair, with hands resting on its back, this time with your left foot on half-toe, right hand on hip (see Position **1**). Push hip out *into* hand, bending right knee. Now! As you *slowly* straighten up, keep weight on right heel, squeeze both buttocks and pull in abdominals (see Position **2**). Once again, you're doing a pelvic tilt. Do 4 sets of 8 reps, alternating sides. Very soon this turns into a jazz dance move. Terrific.

THE BUTT LOVERS HOPSCOTCH

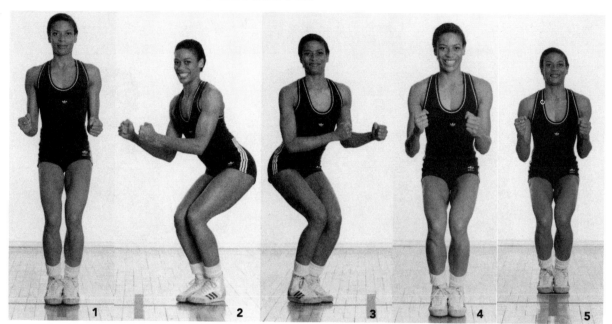

This one is simple—but it works!

From the center point (see Position **1**), jump to the left (see Position **2**), then back to the center. Jump to the right (see Position **3**), then back to the center. Jump forward (see Position **4**), then back to the center. Jump back (see Position **5**), then back to the center.

Too easy? We'll see.

Do 4 sets of 8 reps each of the full series as described above.

THE CHUBBY CHECKERS JUMP TWIST (Come on, baby!)

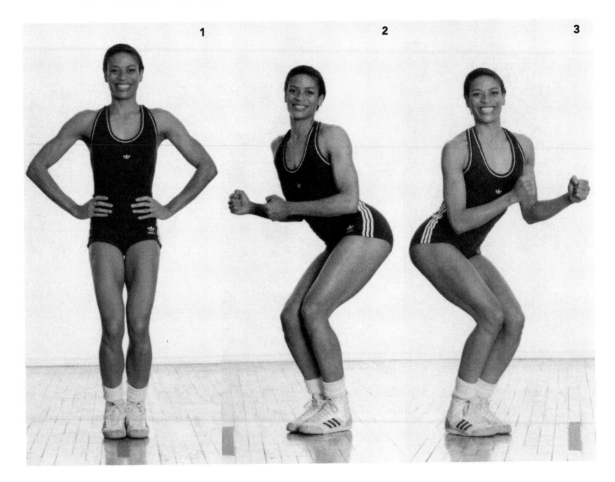

Assume the readiness position with feet together (see Postion **1**). Tighten buttocks, belly button to spine. Jump off the floor, twisting to left (see Position **2**). Now jump and twist to the right (see Position **3**). Continue for 8 counts, 4 sets of 8 reps each.

Checkpoint for Jump Twist

Really push your buttocks to the extreme to right and left.

JAZZ HIP ISOLATION

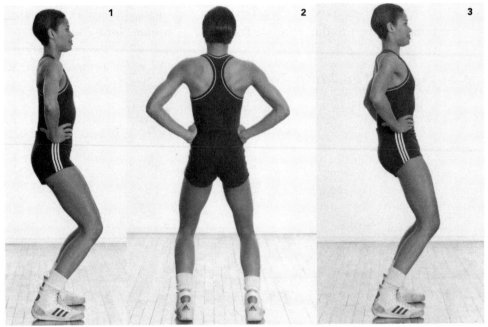

This sounds complicated, but after you do it a couple of times, it's a real rhythmic natural.

Assume the readiness position, with hands on hip joints (see Positions **1** and **2**). Tilt pelvis up and forward by squeezing buttocks and keeping belly button to spine (see Position **3**). Release. Repeat 8 times. Now, keeping shoulders steady, and bending left knee slightly, push hip to right (see Position **4**), return to center, and repeat 8 times. Next, keep belly button to spine, push buttocks backward (see Position **5**), return to center, and repeat 8 times.

Push hip to left (see Position **6**), return to center, and repeat 8 times.
Now put it all together! In rhythm, counting push-two-push-four. Push-two-push-four. Like that!

Push to the front twice, counting four.

Push to the right twice, counting four.

Push to the rear twice, counting four.

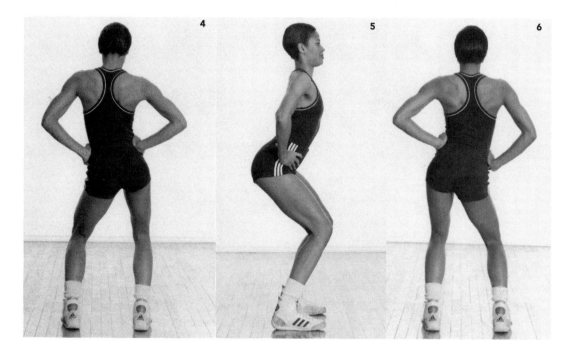

Push to the left twice, counting four.

Do eight reps of this. Then repeat, but to just a 2 count. In other words, push forward, back to center. Push to right, and back to center. Complete the circuit, 8 times.

Finally, incorporate this entire movement into a slow circle, encompassing all four positions, returning to center after each.

Don't get confused by this. Just do it slowly at first, to your own rhythm. You'll soon find yourself doing it through the day. It feels absolutely joyous when you get it down, and it works just fine on the dance floor, too.

Checkpoint for Jazz Hip Isolation

Keep your head and shoulders level and facing forward throughout. Do not let your chest collapse or shoulders shrug up or press forward. But do keep your belly button pressed to your spine, and keep those abs tightened.

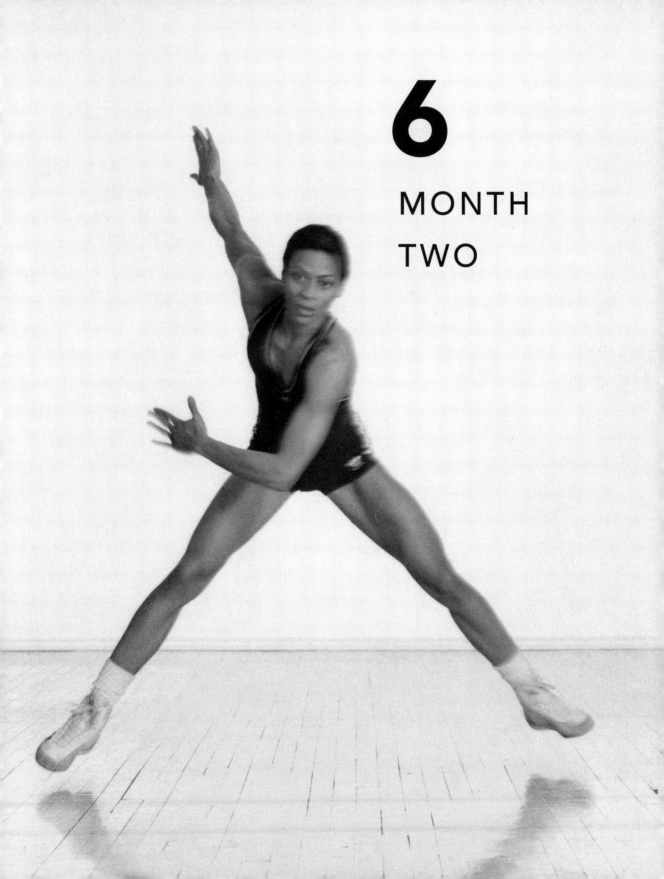

6

MONTH
TWO

Did Those Beginner Weeks Fly or What!

Your body is in much, much better shape than when you began four short weeks ago, and your Gold Medal Butt is already taking shape. But the next four weeks are going to show even greater improvement. The exercises won't be much harder at all, in fact you'll still be doing some of your favorites, with an added twist. As in month one, do as many as possible in thirty minutes, until you can do all twelve. Before you know it, you'll be mastering these as well! You'll need ankle weights for most of the exercises this month. Buy yourself the type where you can add weight in one-pound increments.

Again, remember your breathing. Inhale as you get set; exhale as you exert. Don't forget your abs and trunk strenthening (see Chapter 10). Stretch after your workout (see Chapter 11). And keep up your cardiovascular program!

SEATED STRAIGHT LEG RAISE

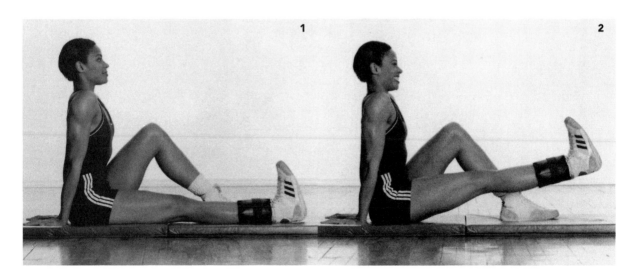

This one is familiar to all fencers. Sit on the floor using your hands for support, left leg bent to chest, right leg extended, right foot flexed (see Position **1**). Lift your right leg, foot flexed, 6 inches off the floor (see Position **2**). Hold for 2 seconds. *Slowly* release. Do 4 sets of 8 reps for each leg. Use 1-pound ankle weights. Increase by 1 pound every fourth workout, up to 10 pounds.

Checkpoint for Straight Leg Raise

Initiate every leg lift from abdominals, do not hyperextend either leg. Keep belly button pressed to spine; keep buttocks squeezed during lift.

ADDUCTION AT 90 DEGREES

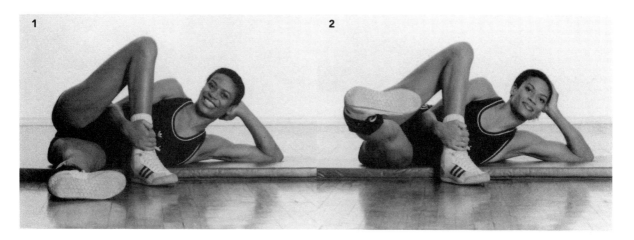

Lie on your left side, with your left leg extended to 3 o'clock and your right leg crossed over left, held by your right hand (see Position **1**). Foot flexed, raise left leg by 12 inches (see Position **2**), hold for 2 seconds. Release and repeat for 8 reps. Lie on right side. Do complete exercise with right leg. Do 4 sets, 8 reps each, alternating sides. Use 1-pound ankle weights. Increase by 1 pound every fourth workout, up to 10 pounds.

HIP EXTENSION

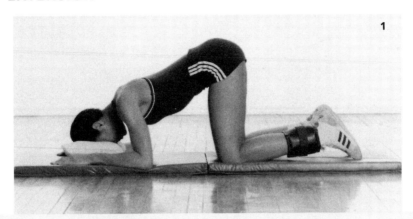

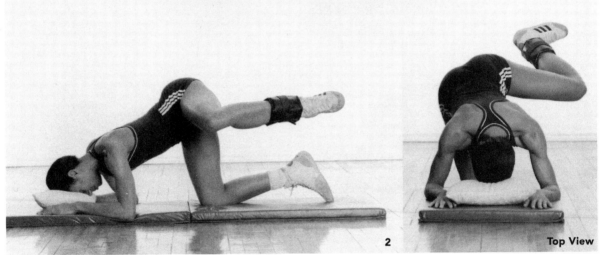

Support yourself on your knees and elbows, hands flat on floor, head resting on pillow (see Position **1**). Flex left foot, raise leg in line with body, approaching a 45-degree angle (see Position **2** and **Top View**). Hold for 2 seconds. *Slowly* release. Do 4 sets of 5 reps for both legs. Use 1-pound ankle weights. Increase by 1 pound every fourth workout, up to 10 pounds.

ABDUCTION AT 90 DEGREES

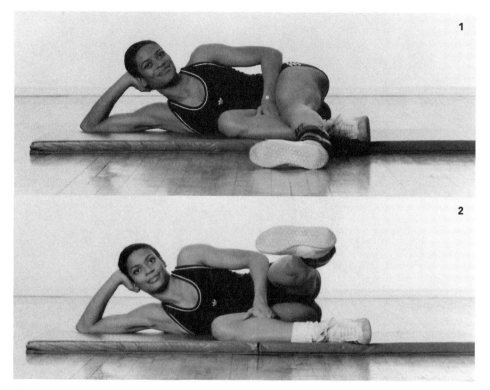

Lie on your right side, head in right hand, with your right leg pulled to chest and your left hand on the floor (see Position **1**). Lift left leg, flexed, 6 to 12 inches (see Position **2**). Hold for a 2 count. Slowly release. Repeat 8 times. Lie on your left side and do the exercise with the right leg. Do 4 sets of 8 reps each, alternating sides. Use 1-pound ankle weights. Increase by 1 pound every fourth workout, up to 10 pounds.

DIAGONAL HIP EXTENSION AT CHAIR

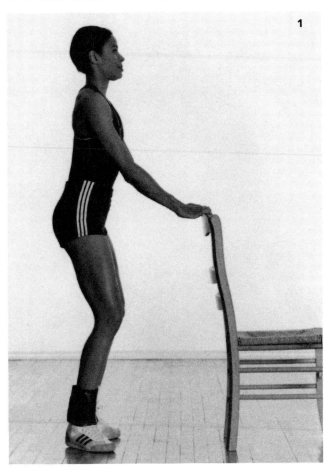

Assume the readiness position, but with feet turned out, and knees slightly bent (see Position **1**). Raise your right leg, foot flexed (see Position **2** and **Back View**). Hold for 2 seconds. Release. Repeat 8 times. Repeat the exercise for left leg. Do 4 sets of 8 reps. Use 1-pound ankle weights. Increase by 1 pound every fourth workout, up to 10 pounds.

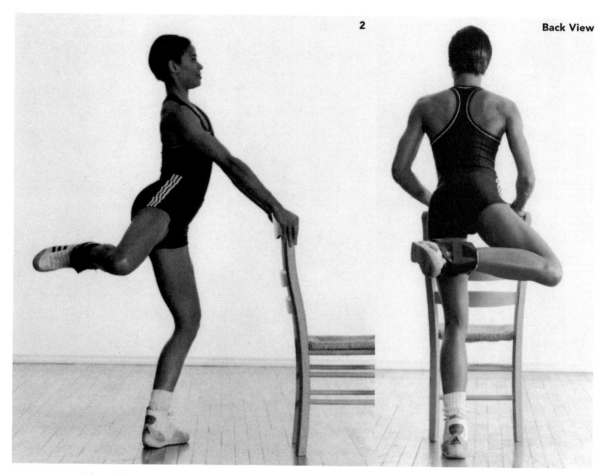

2   **Back View**

Checkpoint for Diagonal Hip Extension

Remember to avoid shoulder elevation during this exercise. Indeed, you
should *feel* your shoulders press downward.

STANDING HIP EXTENSION AT CHAIR

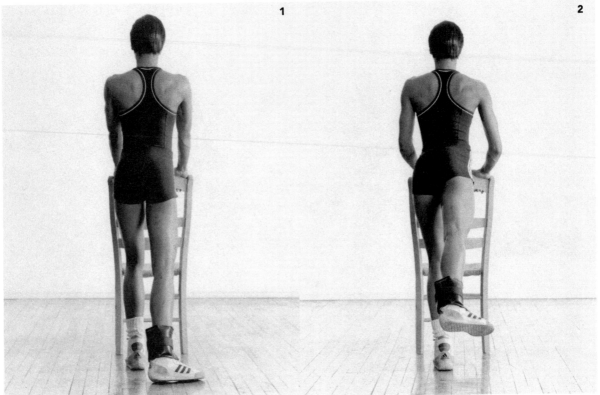

Stand facing the back of the chair, with hands resting on its back, belly button pressed to spine (see Position **1**). Raise your right foot, flexed, 12 inches from the floor (see Position **2**). Hold 2 seconds. Release. Repeat 8 times. Repeat the exercise for each leg. Do 4 sets of 8 reps, each leg. Use 1-pound ankle weights. Increase by 1 pound every fourth workout, up to 10 pounds.

Checkpoint for Standing Hip Extension

To insure that your body is in proper alignment, stand so you *could* raise yourself on the ball of your supporting foot at any time. This will help keep your body from drifting to the right or left.

SINGLE HEEL RAISES

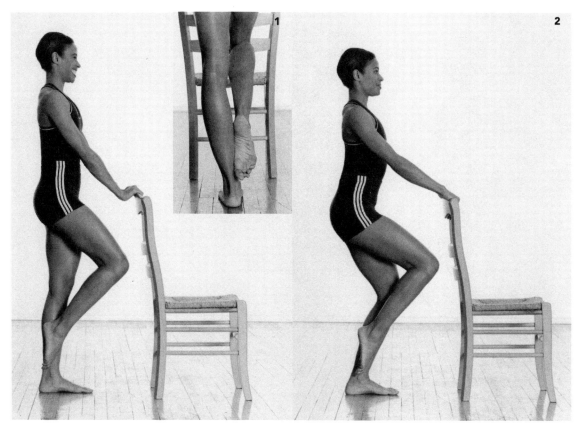

Stand behind a chair, right ankle at left calf (see Position **1** and close-up). Bend left knee without lifting heel from floor (see Position **2**). (This is a pure fencer's move.) Hold for 2 seconds. Straighten up. Now rise on ball of your left foot (see Position **3** and close-up). Hold for 2 seconds, contracting left buttock. Return to first position.

Perform the same exercise with your left ankle at right calf, this time contracting right buttock. Do 4 sets of 8 reps, each leg. Use 1-pound ankle weights. Add 1 pound every fourth workout, up to 10 pounds.

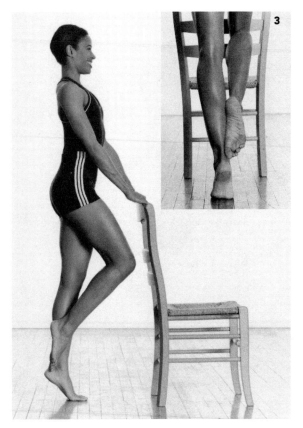

Checkpoint for Single Heel Raises

Be certain to keep your weight on your first two toes when rising to the balls of your feet. Do not let feet turn out as you rise.

CHAIR SQUAT

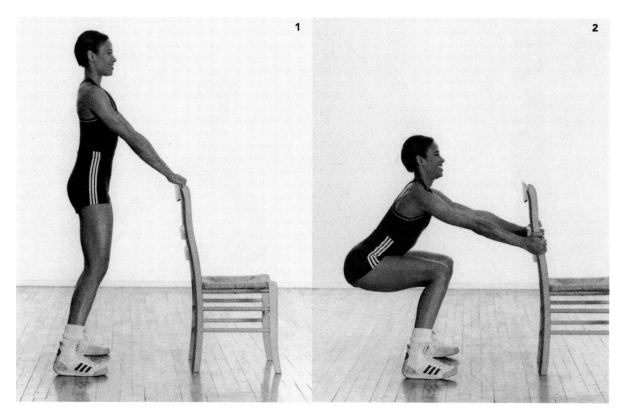

Stand about 12 inches behind a kitchen chair, with your feet flat. Look straight ahead, and press belly button to spine (see Position **1**). Supporting yourself with the chair and keeping your chest high and abdominals tight, push buttocks out as you lean slightly forward to almost form a 90-degree angle (see Position **2**). Hold for a 2 count, then slowly rise, tighten or squeeze glutes as you move. Do 4 sets of 8 reps each. *Note*: On rising, get all the power from your buttocks and lower abdominals. This automatically pushes you into a pelvic tilt. So actually push your hips to the ceiling.

It feels great!

DEAD LIFT WITH CHAIR

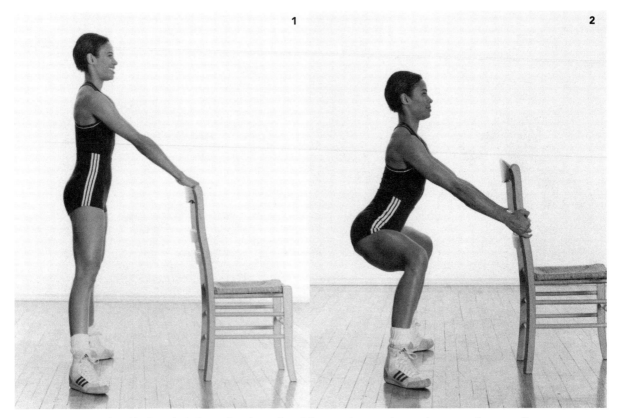

Stand with feet slightly wider than shoulders and turned out about 45 degrees, facing back of chair, with hands resting on its back, (see Position **1**). Push butt backward as knees bend, *keeping weight well back on heels!* Lower yourself to a 90-degree angle (see Position **2**). Hold for a 2 count. As you rise, keep belly button to spine, and thrust your hips toward the ceiling for a pelvic tilt. Do 4 sets of 8 reps each.

Checkpoint for Dead Lift with Chair

Do not try to keep your back straight; let it give a little. Squeeze, tighten, and hold at 2 count.

CHAIR JAZZ SQUAT

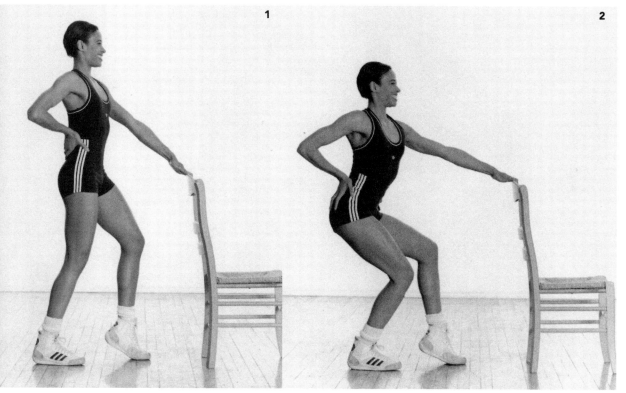

This is a diagonal.

Stand behind the chair, left foot on half-toe, right hand on hip (see Position **1**). Push hip out *into* hand, bending right knee (see Position **2**). Now, as you *slowly* straighten up, keep weight on right heel, squeeze both buttocks and pull in abdominals. Once again, you're doing a pelvic tilt. Do 4 sets of 8 reps, alternating sides.

GRASS DRILLS

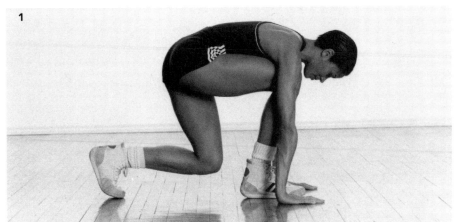

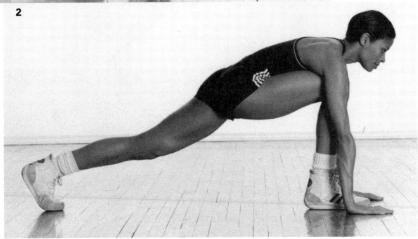

These are fun.

Get on all fours, knees off the floor (see Position **1**). Then switch feet, left and right (see Position **2**). Switch feet 8 times, and do 4 sets. And keep your belly button pressed to the spine.

THE MAJORETTE

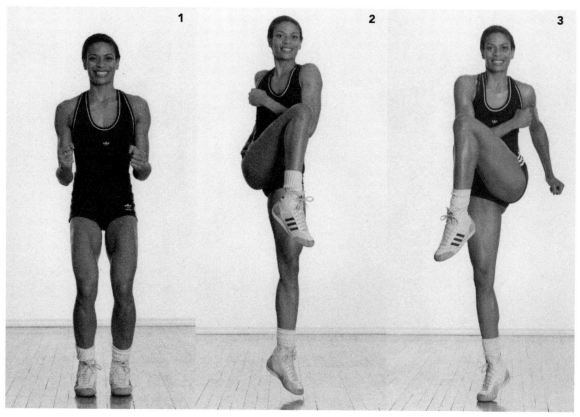

Feel like you did in grade school! Do both.

Assume the readiness position (see Position **1**). Hopping on your left foot, bring your right knee up toward your chest (see Position **2**). Now hop on your right foot, and bring left knee up toward chest (see Position **3**). Do 4 sets of 8 reps each.

Assume the readiness position (see Position **1**). Hopping on your left foot, bring your right knee up toward your chest. Hop on left foot *again*, this time *extending* your right leg (see Position **4**). Do 8 times. Then, hopping on your right foot, bring left knee toward chest, and extend leg (see Position **5**). Do 4 sets of 8 reps.

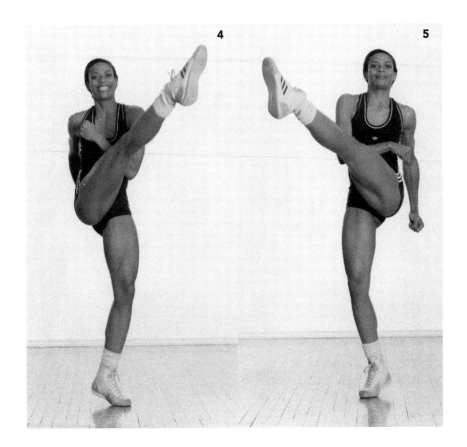

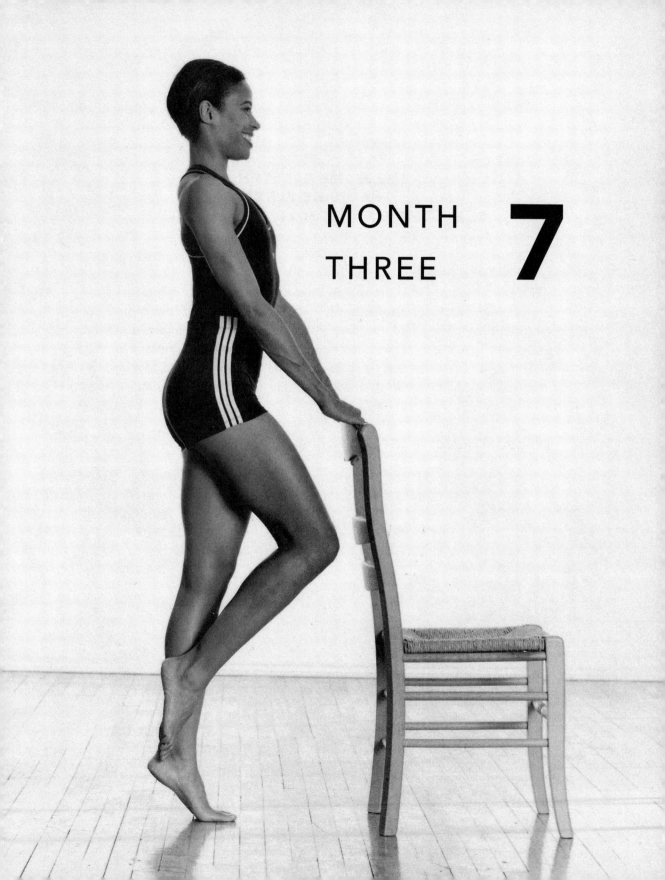

MONTH
THREE

7

THE HOME STRETCH
THE HOME FLEX
THE HOME OF THE GOLD MEDAL BUTT

Look how far you've come.

Don't you feel great? Don't you look great? Aren't you great? You sure are. Because you've proved, to anybody who takes a look, that you're in control of your mind, your body, and your life. So here we go with the advanced moves you're now ready for. Moves that would have been almost impossible two months ago. But moves that you'll now take in stride. (The kind of strutting stride you probably notice in your walk these fine days.) You will continue to use ankle weights.

SEATED STRAIGHT LEG RAISE

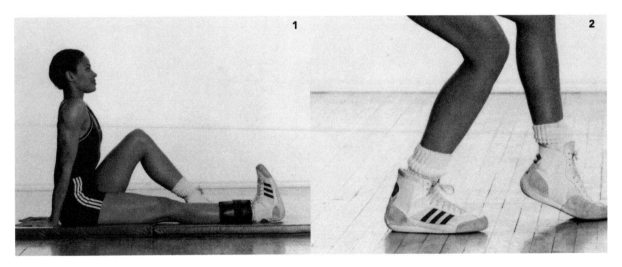

Familiar to all fencers. Sit on the floor using your hands for support, left leg bent to chest, right leg extended, right toe flexed (see Position **1**). Lift your right leg, foot flexed, 6 inches off the floor (see Position **2**). Hold for 2 seconds. *Slowly* release. Do 4 sets of 8 reps for each leg. Use 1-pound ankle weights. Increase by 1 pound every fourth workout, up to 10 pounds.

Checkpoint for Straight Leg Raise

Initiate every leg lift from abdominals, do not hyperextend either leg. Keep belly button pressed to spine; keep buttocks squeezed during lift.

ADDUCTION

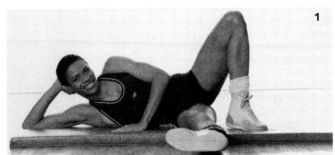

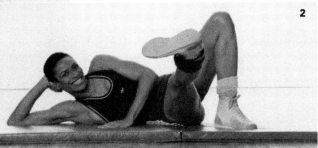

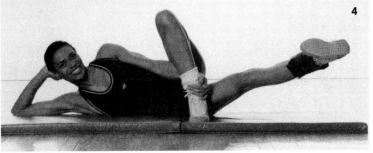

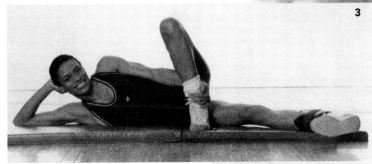

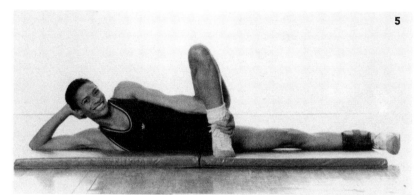

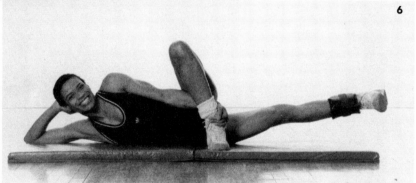

Lie on your right side, with your right leg extended to 3 o'clock and left leg crossed over right, held by left hand (see Position **1**). Raise right leg 12 inches, and hold for 2 seconds (see Position **2**). Release. Repeat for 8 reps.

Lie on your left side and do the complete exercise with the left leg. Do 4 sets of 8 reps each, alternating sides.

Repeat the exercise at 45 degrees (see Positions **3** and **4**) and at 0 degrees (see Positions **5** and **6**).

Use 1-pound ankle weights. Add 1 pound every fourth workout, up to 10 pounds.

ABDUCTION

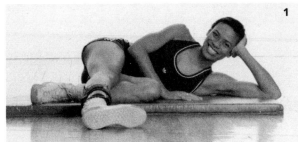

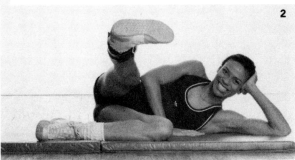

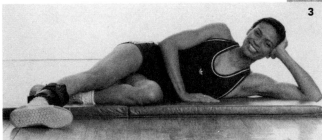

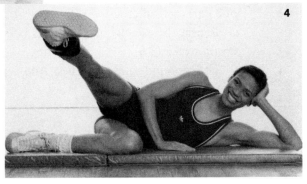

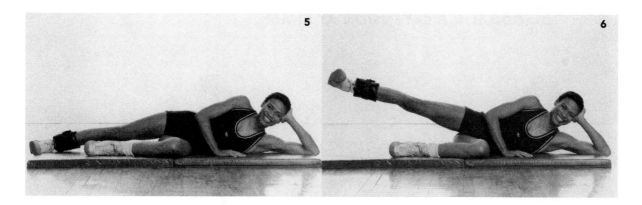

Lie on your left side, head in left hand, with left leg pulled to chest with right hand (see Position **1**). Lift right leg, flexed, 6 to 12 inches (see Position **2**). Hold for a 2 count. Slowly release. Repeat 8 times. Lie on your right side, and do the exercise with your left leg. Do 4 sets of 8 reps, alternating sides. Repeat exercises at 45 degrees (see Positions **3** and **4**) and 0 degrees (see Positions **5** and **6**).

Use 1-pound ankle weights. Add 1 pound every fourth workout, up to 10 pounds.

DIAGONAL HIP EXTENSION AT CHAIR

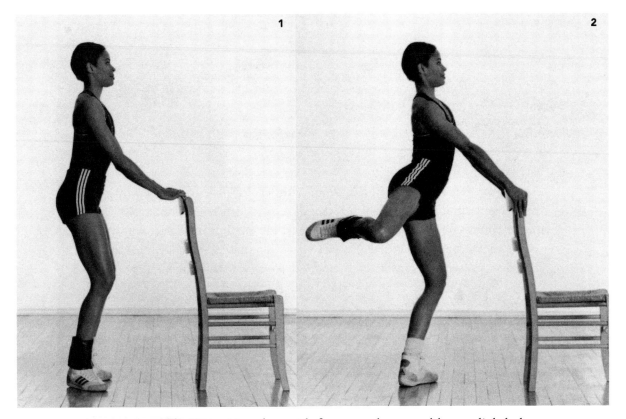

Assume the readiness position, but with feet turned out, and knees slightly bent (see Position **1**). Raise your right leg, foot flexed (see Position **2** and **Back View**). Hold for 2 seconds. Release. Repeat 8 times.

Repeat the exercise for the left leg. Do 4 sets of 8 reps, alternating legs. Use 1-pound ankle weights. Increase by 1 pound every fourth workout, up to 10 pounds.

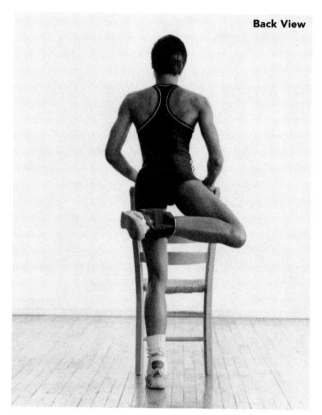

Back View

Checkpoint for Diagonal Hip Extension at Chair

Remember to avoid shoulder elevation during this exercise. Indeed, you should *feel* your shoulders press downward.

SINGLE HEEL RAISES

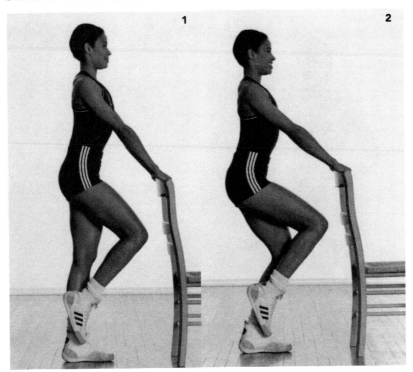

Stand behind chair, with your right ankle at left calf (see Position **1**). Bend your left knee without lifting the foot from the floor (see Position **2**). (This is a pure fencer's move.) Hold for 2 count. Straighten up. Now rise on the ball of your left foot, contracting left buttock (see Position **3**). Hold for a 2 count. Return to the first position.

Perform the same exercise with your left ankle at left calf, this time contracting right buttock. Do 4 sets of 8 reps, each leg. Use 1-pound ankle weights. Increase by 1 pound every fourth workout, up to 10 pounds.

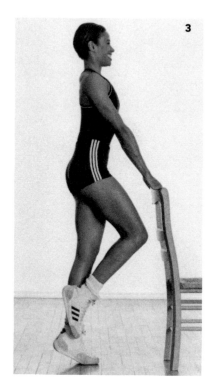

Checkpoint for Single Heel Raises

Be certain to keep your weight on your first two toes when rising to balls of your feet. Do not let your feet turn out as you rise.

SQUATS

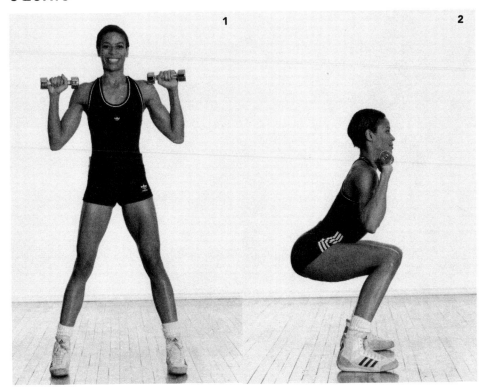

Assume the readiness position (see Position **1**). (You can adjust your feet outward to a 45-degree angle, which allows a greater depth of squat, but at the same time takes pressure off the quadriceps, slimming the thigh.) With slightly bent knees, push buttocks out at waist until back is perpendicular to the floor (see Position **2**). Keeping belly button pressed to spine, shoulders back. Hold for 2 seconds. Come back to Position 1, but as you come back erect, get all the power for that move by squeezing the buttocks, using a pelvic tilt to assume Position **1**. Do 4 sets of 8 reps each. Use 5-pound dumbbells to start.

Checkpoint for Squats

Keep your weight well back on your heels throughout. This keeps pressure off quads that keeps thighs slim. And never let your knees move forward over the toes.

DEAD LIFT

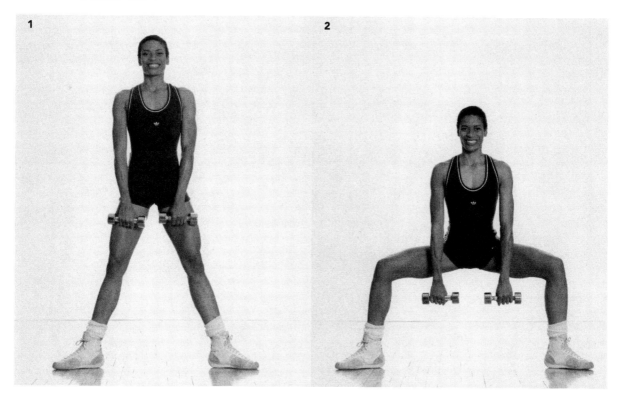

With your feet comfortably turned out, hold 5-pound dumbbells with arms extended downward, in front of body (see Position **1**). Push buttocks out as you dip to 90 degrees, chest high, belly button to spine, back tipped forward (see Position **2**). Hold for a 2 count. Return to Position **1**. Do 5 sets of 5 reps each.

Checkpoint for Dead Lift

Keep your knees turned outward over toes, don't let those thighs turn inward. This helps keep thighs thinner!

FRONT LUNGE AT CHAIR

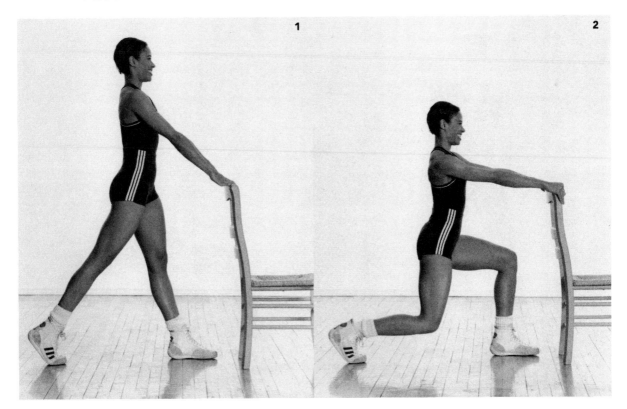

A pure fencing movement. Stand at chair, right leg back, on half-toe, facing straight ahead, with belly button pressed to spine (see Position **1**). Kneel until your right knee touches the floor (or comes as close as possible—you'll improve), contracting buttocks *and* abdominals at the same time (see Position **2** and **Back View**). Hold for a 2 count. As you rise up, supported by the the chair, keep your chest high, belly button to spine, and develop your pelvic tilt. Do 4 sets of 3 reps each, alternating sides.

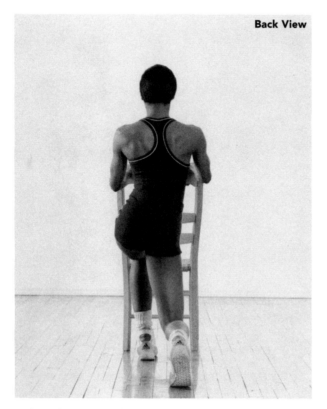

Back View

Checkpoint for Front Lunge at Chair

As you bend, take care not to let your front knee extend over your toe. To avoid that, simply extend your other leg farther back. And *use your chair for support!*

SIDE LUNGE AT CHAIR

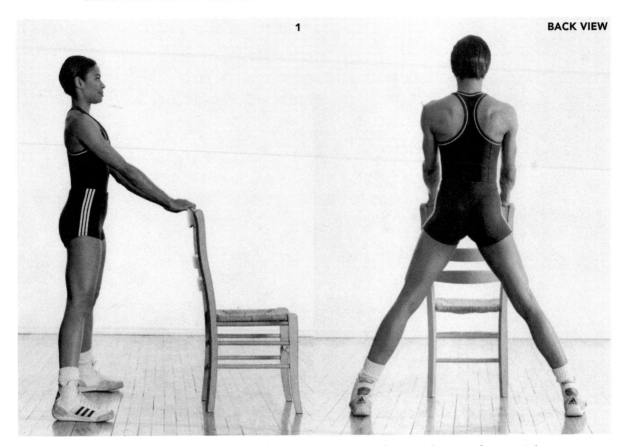

A fencing move that you will love. Stand at the chair with your feet straight ahead and wider than your shoulders (see Position **1** and **Back View**). Push right buttock back and down, bending your right knee as far as possible. Keep left leg straight. You're almost doing a one-legged squat (see Position **2** and **Back View**). Hold for 2 seconds. Squeeze or tighten both lower extremeties as you move. Stand. Repeat 8 times. Do 4 sets of 8 reps, each leg.

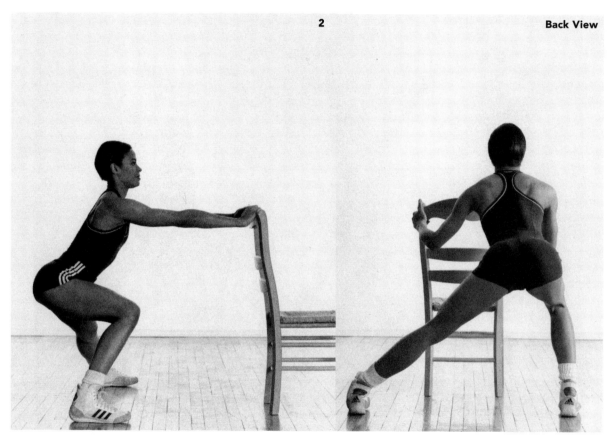

Checkpoint for Side Lunge at Chair

Keep feet flat. Keep abdominals tight, and belly button pressed to spine. Don't let your knees extend beyond your toes and stay back on your heels.

THE WINDMILL LUNGE

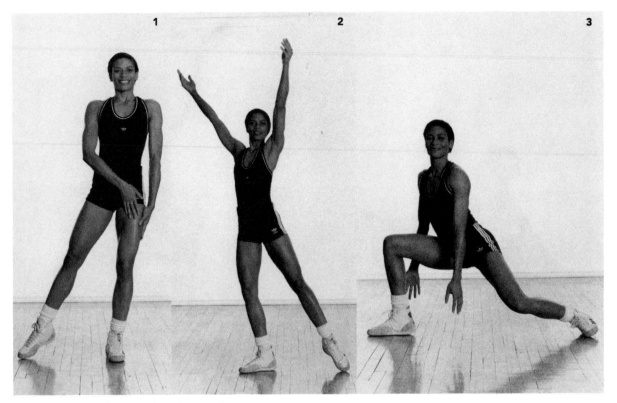

Much easier than it sounds.

Assume the readiness position, with both arms on left side at hip (see Position **1**). Now fan arms over your head (see Position **2**), all the way down to touch the floor on the right side (see Position **3**). Fan arms up from floor, all the way to touch the floor on left side (see Positions **4** and **5**).

Now, do the same, but increase the speed slightly, and as speed increases, do slight jump, switching weight from one leg to another. If your legs are very long or you are not stretched out enough, go only as far as you can without straining.

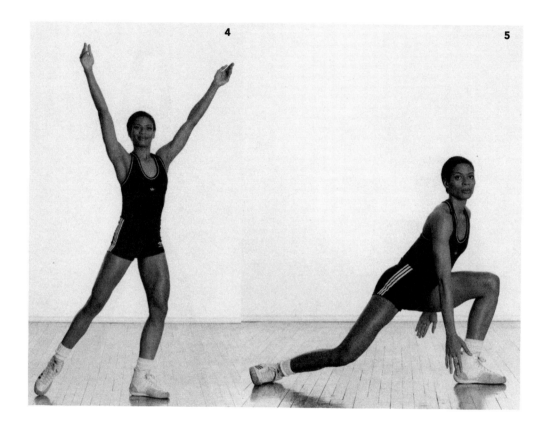

SQUAT JUMPS (with a Difference)

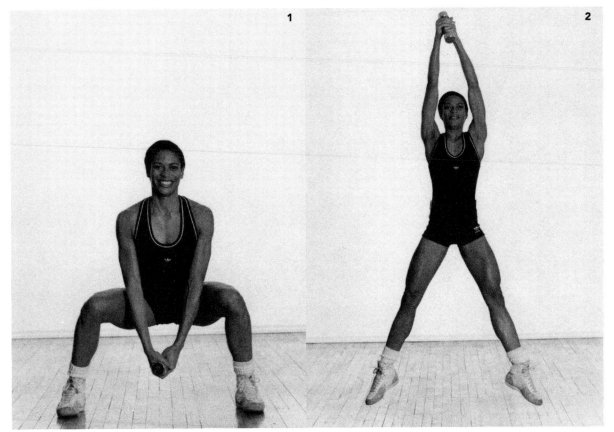

Start in the dead lift position, hands clasped at crotch (see Position **1**). Leap up, legs out, hands flung high (see Position **2**). Repeat 8 times. Do 4 complete sets. Flinging your hands high helps you jump higher, and stretches your buttocks more. Keeping your eyes on your upstretched hands (like you're going for a rebound) helps you land softer.

Checkpoint for Squat Jumps

When jumping, lock your elbows. This keeps your rib cage over your pelvis, and helps strengthen your abdominals.

RUNNING-IN-PLACE LUNGE

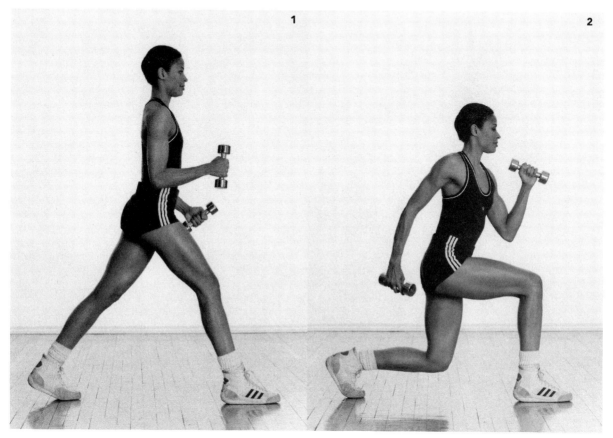

A pure fencing maneuver. Stand with your feet in the lunge position, and your back foot on half-toe (see Position **1**). Bend forward knee to form a nearly 90-degree angle (see Position **2**). Now, swinging arms, switch back foot to front position. Repeat, back and forth, in place, swinging arms vigorously, for 4 sets of 8 jumps each. Use 5-pound dumbbells to start. Repeat on opposite side.

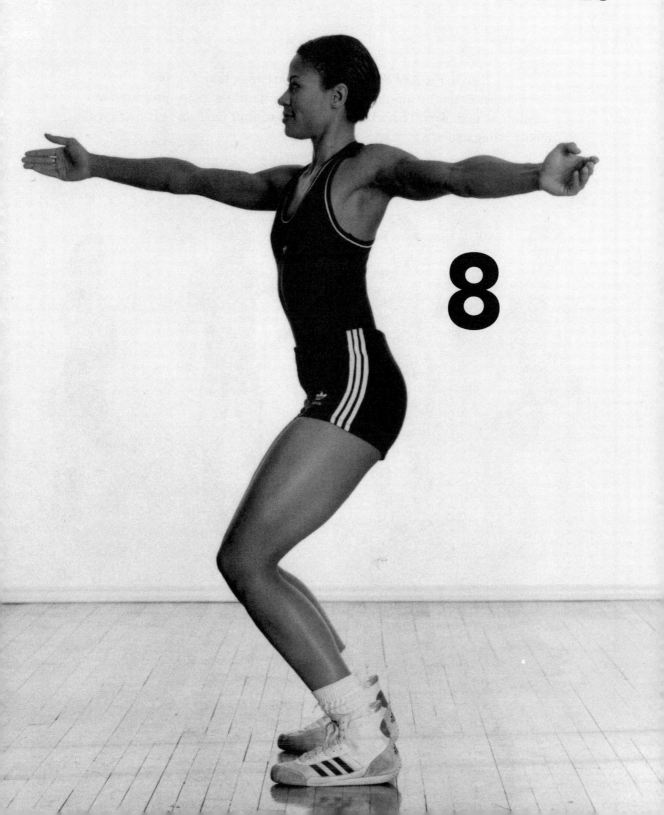

Exercises to Add Some Spice and Variety to Your Routines

These exercises can be substituted for any exercise in the home program (one substitution each day). They can also be added to your program to deliver even more striking results.

THE FENCER CONDENSOR

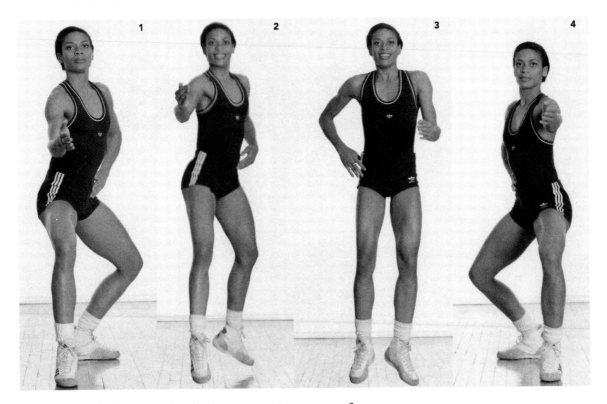

In which you pack tight butt power into our perfect movement.

Assume the classic fencer's posture: back foot turned out, front foot pointed forward, with lead arm extended as if holding a sword (see Position **1**). Jump into the air, land in place in a mirror position (see Positions **2**, **3**, and **4**). Do 4 sets of 8 reps, for each leg.

CLEAN AND JERK

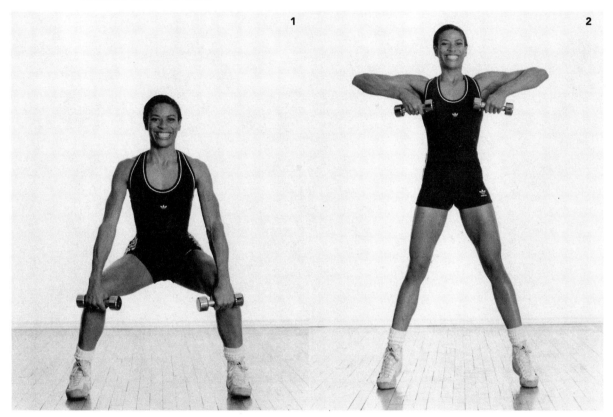

A move all fencers work. Assume the readiness position: knees bent, weight on heels, arms extended downward, 5-pound dumbbells in hands (see Position **1**). Using your butt, push yourself up, raising hands to chest, pushing yourself up on toes (see Position **2**). Hold for a 2 count. Walk through this exercise to get the rhythm of it. Then do 4 sets of 8 reps each.

Take the time to learn this exercise well. It is very important, and works its magic powerfully on your Gold Medal Butt.

LUNGE JUMPS

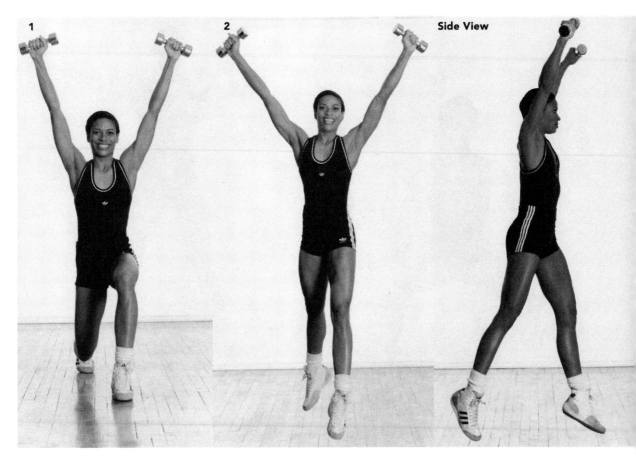

Stand with arms raised, right foot 2 feet to the rear, on ball of foot (see Position **1**). Leap up to your limit (see Position **2** and **Side View**) and land in place, in the same position as Position **1**.

The higher you go, the better for the butt. This is really a great stretcher. Do 4 sets of 8 reps, each side.

SKIPPING—BIG TIME!

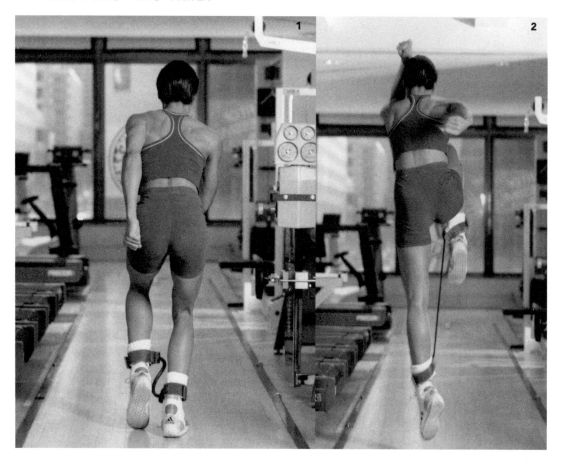

Stand in the lunge jump position (see Position **1**). Now skip in place. (But no kid stuff!)

Bring your knees up as high as possible, flinging your arms high (see Position **2**). Knees up? Higher! Higher!

Sharon is wearing a Sidewinder band, which this exercise can be done with to provide extra resistance and a more rigorous workout.

Do 4 sets of 8 reps, each side.

SKATE JUMP

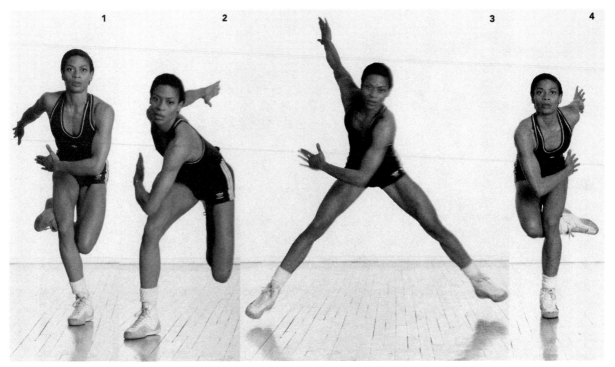

Stand on your right leg (see Position **1**). Jump to the left as far as possible, and land on your left leg (see Positions **2**, **3**, and **4**). Swinging your arms, as pictured, helps you keep your balance. Do 4 sets of 8 reps, each leg.

WALL SITTING

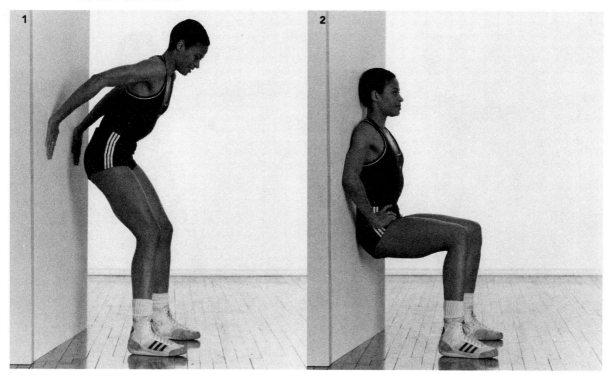

This one's a little tougher than it looks.

Stand at wall, feet straight ahead, heels two feet from wall. Ease into a sitting position with your back against the wall (see Positions **1** and **2**). Hold for 15 seconds, butt contracted. Stand, shake out legs and arms. Repeat 4 more times.

DIAGONALS FOR HIPS

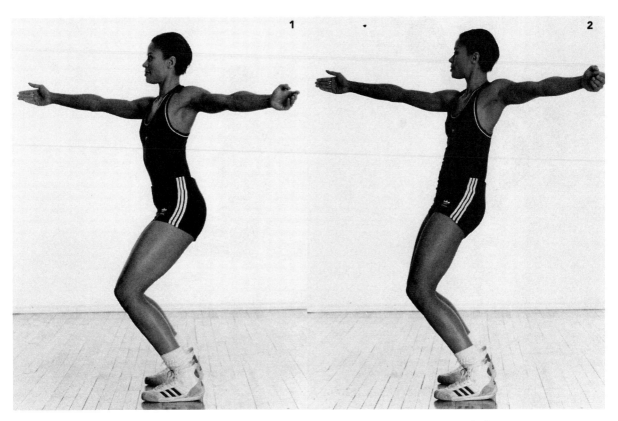

Assume the readiness position, with head facing 12 noon, arms extended to 5 past 12 and 25 to 12 (see Position **1**). Now lift your right hip to follow the line of your right arm (see Position **2**). Return. Now lift your left hip back to follow the line of your left arm (see Position **3**). Return. Do 8 reps.

Now put your left arm at 5 to 12 and right arm at 25 past. Lift your left hip to follow left arm; right hip to follow right arm back. Repeat 8 times. Do total of 4 sets of 8 reps each, in both time zones.

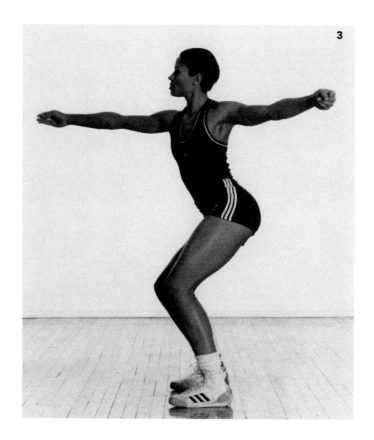

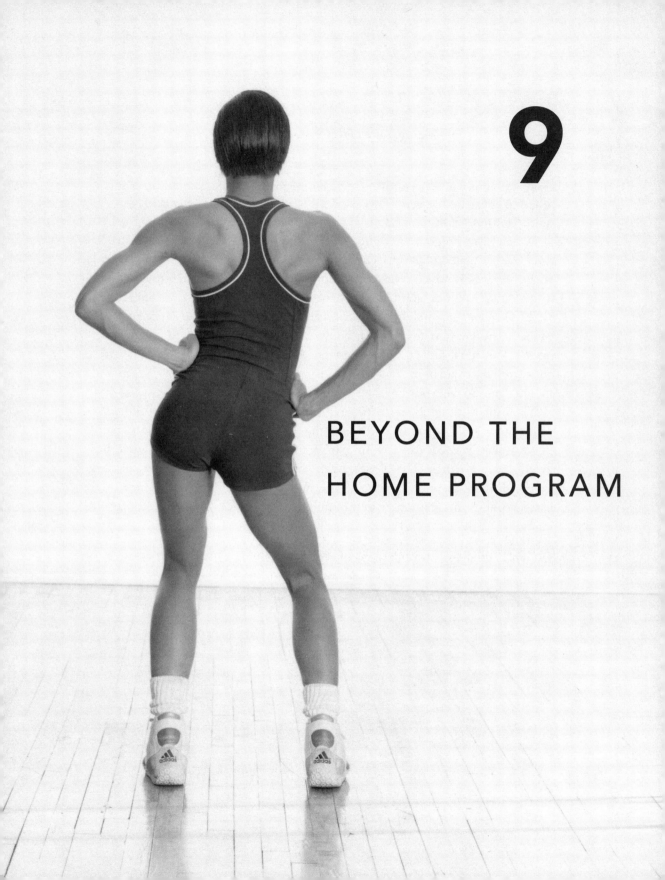

9

BEYOND THE
HOME PROGRAM

Enhancing Your Gold Medal Butt at the Gym

Congratulations! You've completed the Home Program. You should be very proud of yourself—we certainly are proud of you. Now, if you want to continue your pursuit of the perfect butt, you'll want to start our Gym Program.

Why a Gym Program? Weights get results faster and are more pinpointed at trouble areas than any other technique. That's because weights can simply (and safely) *overload* a muscle. This temporary overload jolts a muscle into attention, which actually pumps blood and nutrients into it and speeds up development.

Weights, and *only* weights, can so swiftly give you a sense of balance and help you identify, once and for all, your body's center. It's always located around your middle, and you'll find it for one very good reason: You *can't* use weights without becoming aware of it.

You'll see. So will your butt.

There are three levels to the program: Intermediate, Advanced, and Elite. As you advance, feel free to mix and match the exercises to keep your interest up.

Reminder: Please speak to your gym's trainer before starting this or any other weight-based program. They'll work with you on determining which weights to start with, how to properly execute the movements, when to graduate to the next level of the program, how to mix and match exercises, and help you prevent injury.

INTERMEDIATE

TRU SQUAT

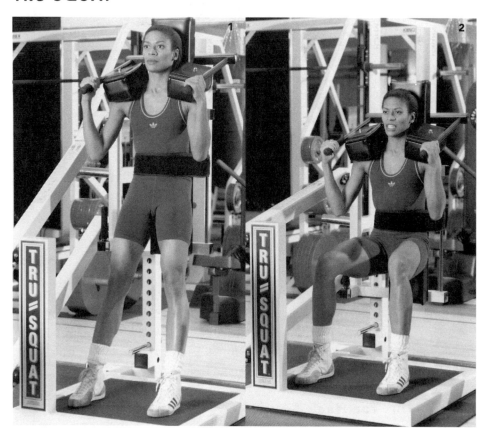

Adjust the machine to the proper height and adjust the Velcro belt. Press shoulder pads slightly up, tense body, and release safety (see Position **1**). Stand with your feet shoulder-width apart, about 12 inches forward of your hips. Lower the machine slowly to a 90-degree position (see Position **2**). Hold for a 2 count and push back up slowly from the heels. Repeat. Do 4 sets of 10 reps.

HACK SQUAT

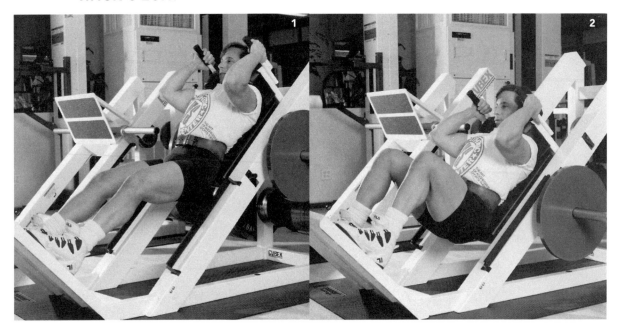

Lie against body pad, shoulders tight against pads, feet shoulder-width apart (see Position **1**). Lower the weight by bending your knees, *always* focusing pressure through your heels (see Position **2**). This directs all results to work on your improving butt. Do 4 sets of 10 reps. (No, your eyes aren't playing tricks. The model is Gary—we decided to give Sharon a break!)

Checkpoint for Hack Squat

Keep abdominals under tight control, belly button to spine.

HORIZONTAL LEG PRESS

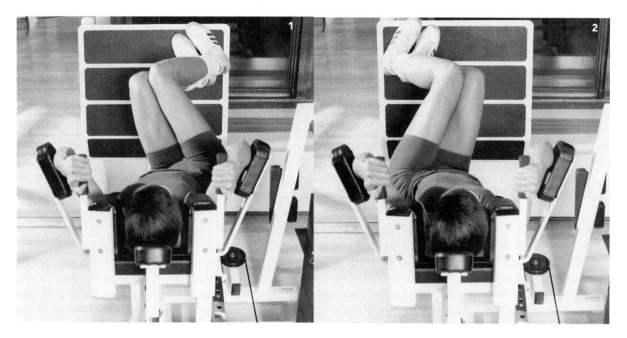

Set the seat at its lowest level. Place your feet together at a 45-degree angle in the upper right corner of the platform (see Position **1**). Focusing your power through your heels, belly button pressed to spine, press out until your legs are fully extended. Do the left side, too (see Position **2**). Do 4 sets of 10 reps.

Checkpoint for Horizontal Leg Press

Extend your legs, yes, but don't lock your knees. That would cause kneecap compression, which could stretch ligaments, a no no!

VERTICAL LEG PRESS

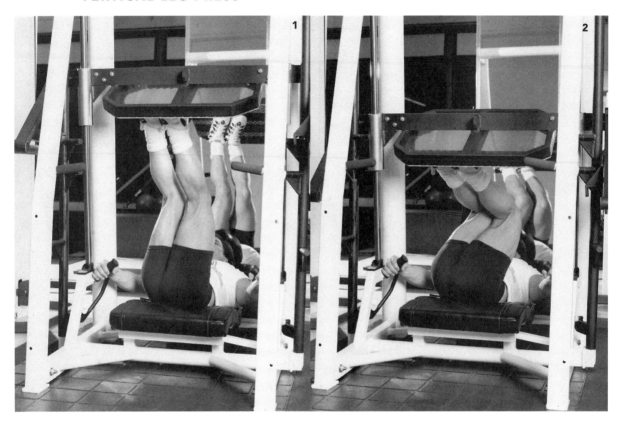

Lie with your neck comfortably on cushion, and your feet on platform, close together at a 45-degree angle. Release safety lever, tensing entire body to accept the weight (see Position **1**). Now lower knees to chest (see Position **2**). Your feet should remain flat throughout but get all resistance through heels. (Feeling effort through heels in all exercises helps make thighs thinner and develops the gluteals.) Do both sides. Do 4 sets of 10 reps.

ABDUCTION ON THE BODY MASTER

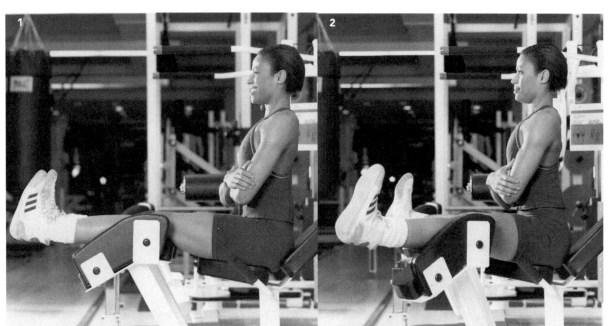

Assume a sitting position, erect, feet flexed back, knees straight (see Position **1**). Press out as far as your legs can go (see Position **2**). (Don't worry, you'll get better and better.) Hold for 2 seconds.

Do 1 set of 15 reps. Then immediately do another set of 15 reps with feet unflexed and knees bent. Repeat for 4 sets total.

Checkpoint for Abduction on the Body Master

Spread legs equally, favoring neither side. This develops the long muscles on the side of the leg that give shape to buttocks.

SUPINE LEG EXTENSION WITH CABLE

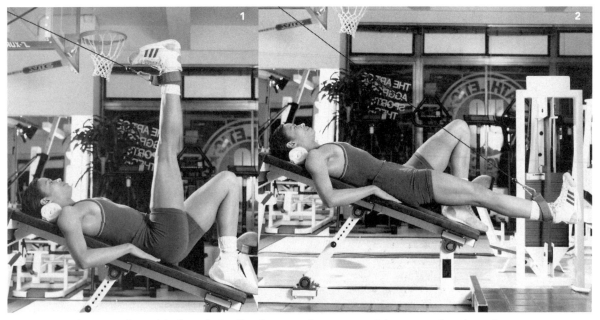

On an adjustable bench inclined to 45 degrees, position your head at the top, supported by a towel roll. Lying flat on your back, attach the cable to the right ankle. With the left knee bent up to 45 degrees, keep the left foot firmly on the bench for balance.

Allow the straight right leg to be drawn up by the cable to almost 90 degrees (see Position **1**). Pause 2 seconds. Push leg slowly down to the bench (see Position **2**). Pause 2 seconds. Repeat 8 times, alternating legs. Do 4 sets of 10 reps.

SEATED LEG CURL

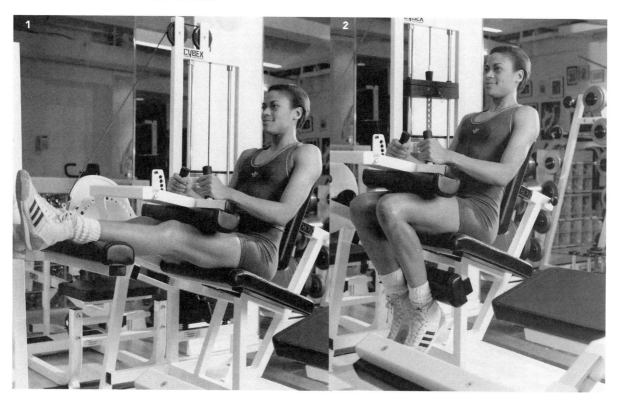

Sit with knee joint lined up with axis on machine. Place foot pad at comfortable position, legs straight (see Position **1**). Lower feet, relaxed, all the way down, while exhaling (see Position **2**). Hold for 2 seconds. Squeeze. Release. Do 4 sets of 10 reps.

HIP EXTENSION WITH KNEES FLEXED

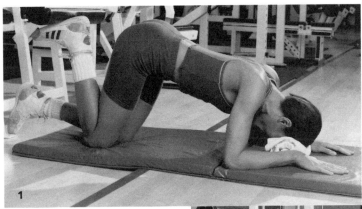

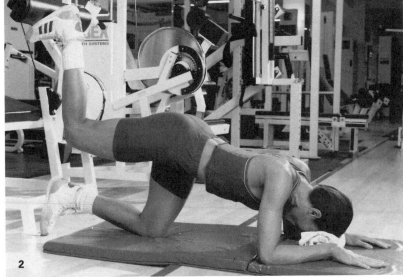

Get down on all fours, in front of prone leg curl machine, kneeling on mat. Place your head on the mat, with your weight resting on forearms and knees. Lift right foot to pad (see Position **1**). Now push your hip to elevate your foot (see Position **2**). (Do not straighten the leg—extend the hip. You'll feel it when it's happening right.) Do 4 sets of 10 reps.

FROGGIES (or Prone Leg Curl)

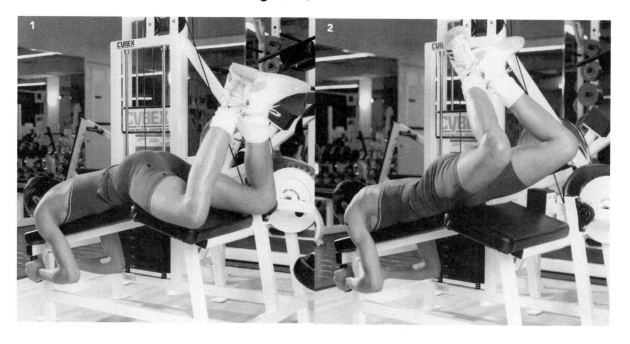

Lie face down, knees bent at 90 degrees and slightly off pad, lined up with joint axis of machine (see Position **1**). Lift legs up till body is level (see Position **2**). Keep feet relaxed, no tension. Press torso into the pad, performing pelvic tilt. Hold for 2 seconds, keeping abs tight, and release. Do 4 sets of 10 reps.

NORDIC-STYLE SKI MACHINE

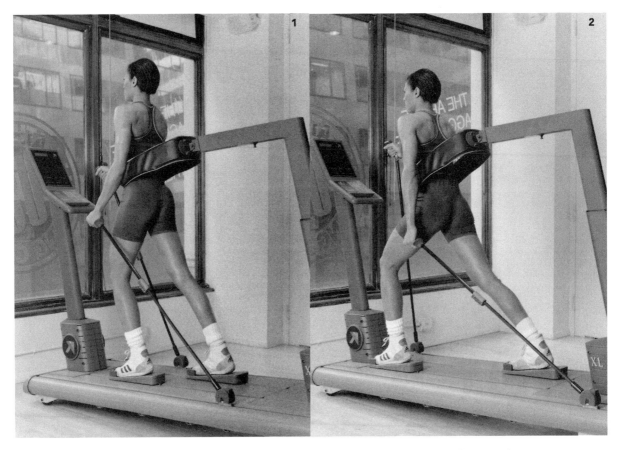

This is Gary's fast-working variation: *Elevate* the rear of the machine with a 6-inch thick wood block. Then perform the regulation cross country ski maneuver (see Positions **1** and **2**). Perform four 30-second sprints.

ADVANCED

SQUATS

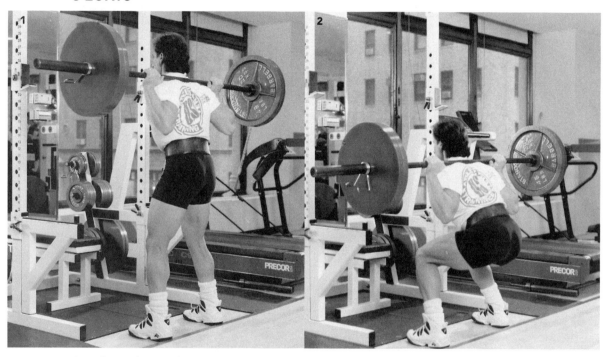

Stand in the readiness position, bar across shoulders. Tense body to accept weight (see Position **1**). Now push your buttocks out as you squat. (That's why their called squats, get it?) It's important to keep your belly button pressed against your spine, chest high, as you lower to a near sitting position. Keep your weight focused through your heels with back tilted slightly forward (see Position **2**.) Hold for a 2 count (one Guerriero, two Guerriero), then return to standing position. Do 5 sets of 5 reps.

DEAD LIFT

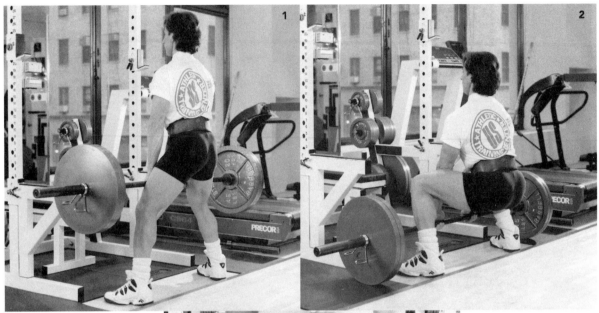

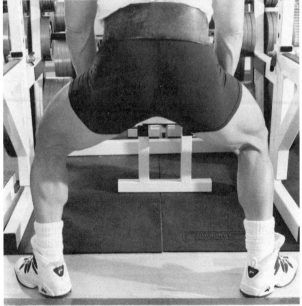

With your feet comfortably turned out (see close-up), hold the bar with your arms extended downward, in front of body (see Position **1**). Push buttocks out as you dip to 90 degrees. (see Position **2**). Keep chest high, belly button to spine, back tipped slightly forward. Hold for 2 seconds and squeeze legs as you return to starting position. Do 5 sets, 5 reps.

Checkpoint for Dead Lifts

Keep knees turned outward, don't extend over toes. Don't let those inner thighs turn inward. This helps keep thighs thinner! When returning to the erect position, after a 2 count, keep buttocks squeezed tight and keep pelvis tipped forward.

FRONT LUNGES

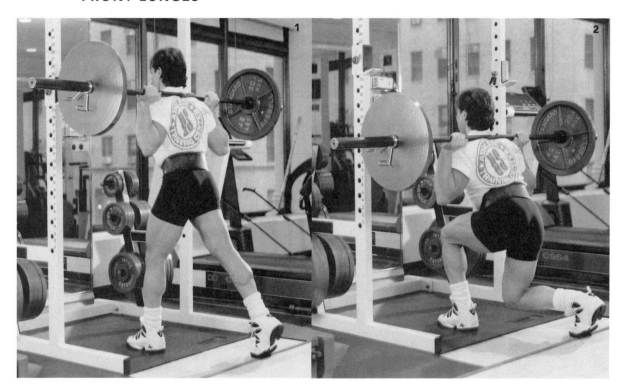

Get positioned with the bar on your shoulders and your right foot back, kneeling on half-toe (see Position **1**). Dip right knee to about 90 degrees, chest high, belly button to spine (see Position **2**). As you kneel, turn left hip to side and slightly back. As you'll feel, this becomes a jazz-move. Do 4 sets of 8 reps for each side.

SIDE LUNGES

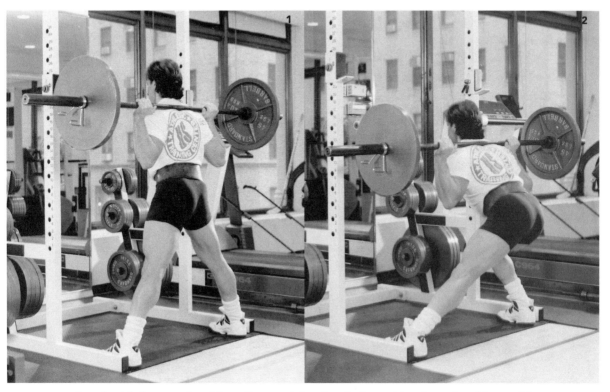

Stand with bar on shoulders, feet straight ahead, feet wider than shoulder width (see Position **1**). Ride hip backward as if you were sitting on a chair placed to one side (see Position **2**). Hold at bottom of movement. Keep chest high, let back curve slightly forward. Do 4 sets of 8 reps, each side.

NAUTILUS SKATE MACHINE

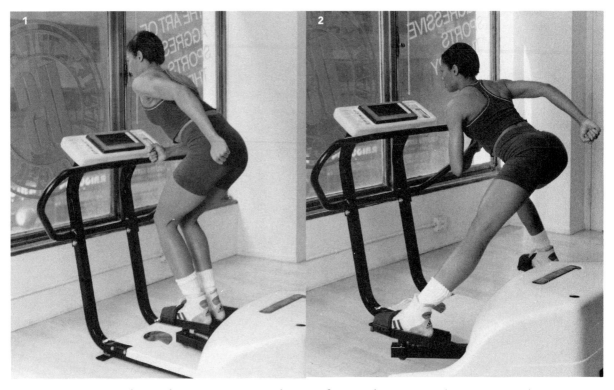

Assume the readiness position, with your feet in the stirrups (see Position **1**). Push out with your right leg, come back to center, then push out with left leg and come back to center (see Position **2**). This is very similar to roller skating, so try it a few times till you get the rhythm down. Then do four 30-second sprints.

ELITE

MODIFIED FRONT LUNGES

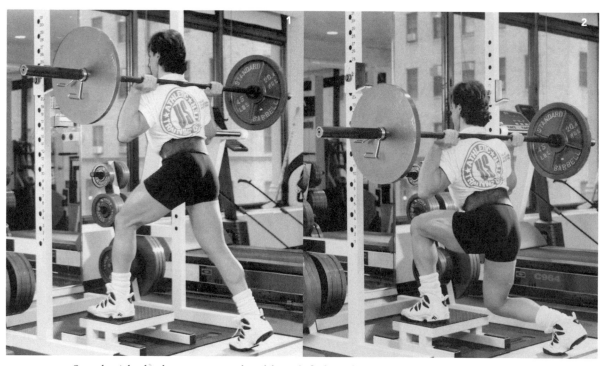

Stand with the bar on your shoulders, left foot forward on raised platform, and right foot back, kneeling on half-toe (see Position **1**). Dip left knee to 90 degrees, keeping chest high and belly button to spine (see Position **2**). As you kneel, turn left hip slightly to side and back. Do 4 sets of 8 reps, each side.

MODIFIED SIDE LUNGES

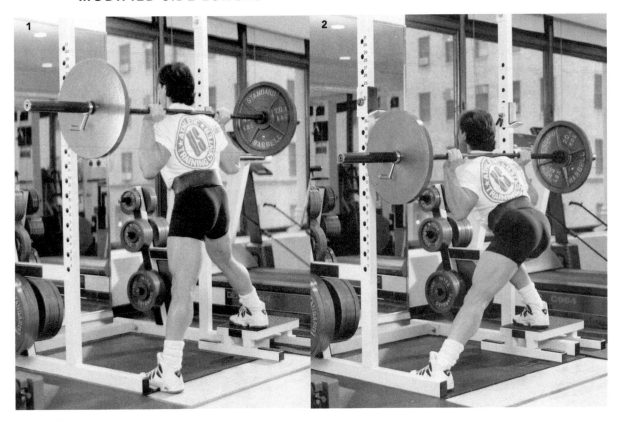

Stand with the bar on your shoulders, left foot planted, right foot on platform on same side (see Position **1**). Ride hip backward almost as if sitting on a chair placed to the right. Keep chest high, and let back curve slightly forward. Hold at bottom of movement (see Position **2**). Feel that tug in your butt? Good! Do 4 sets of 8 reps, each side.

CLEAN AND JERK

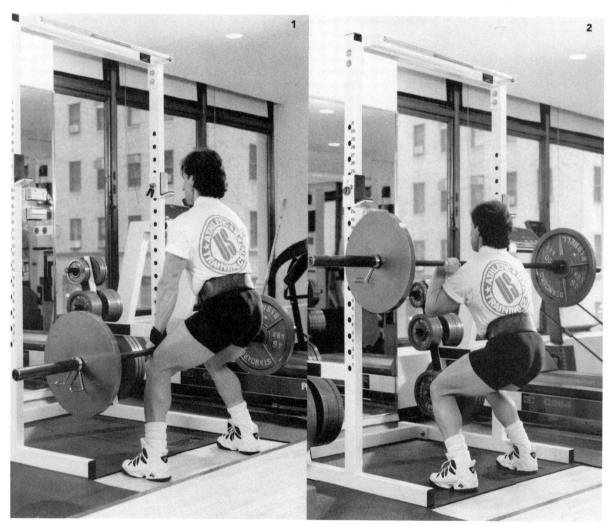

(Fencers *love* this.) We recommend a weight belt for this exercise, to help protect your back. Stand with legs apart, slightly wider than shoulder width. Lift the barbell to knee height, using your butt and legs—not your back (see Position **1**)! Lift to shoulder height, flexing legs (see Position **2**). Bringing right leg back to

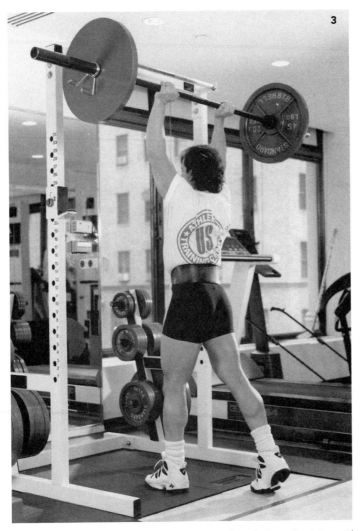

half-toe, push the barbell over your head (see Position **3**). Walk through this exercise to get the rhythm. Then do 4 sets of 8 reps each. Take the time to do this well. It works magic on your Gold Medal Butt.

STANDING LEG CURL

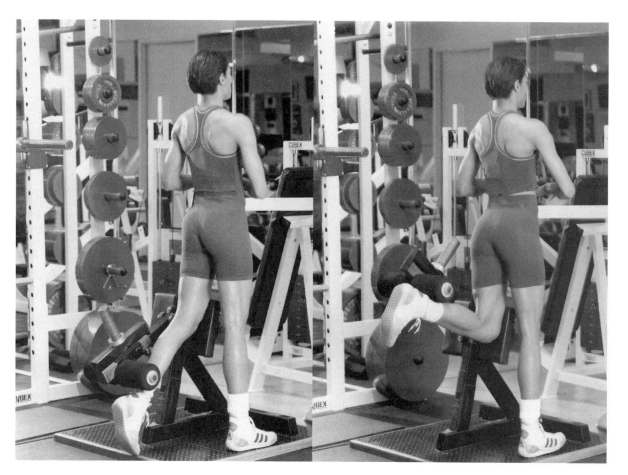

Stand at the machine and *lean into* the pad, with your right foot forward, left thigh and buttocks on pad, and abs *tight* (see Position **1**). Raise left leg to 90 degrees (see Position **2**). Hold for a 2 count. Release. Repeat for right leg. Do 2 sets of 10 reps, each leg.

SIDE-TO-SIDE SLIDE

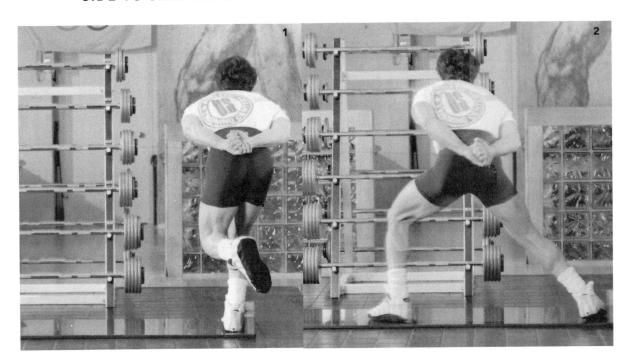

Start in a skating position: left leg bent 45-degrees (off the floor), right leg bent slightly. Both arms are set parallel, gently pointing upward right (see Position **1**). As the left leg moves toward the floor, push with the right leg as the arms swing—everything slides left (see Position **2**).

It's our only free ride, so enjoy it! Reverse the action without stopping. Repeat 8 times.

ONE LEG SQUAT ON GRAVITY-ASSISTED DIP MACHINE

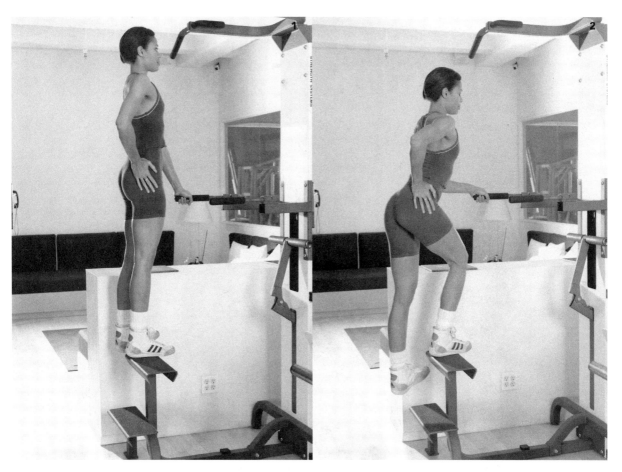

Mount the platform. Place right hand on right hip, left hand on grip (see Position **1**). Dip down on right leg pushing hip into hand as close to 90 degrees as possible (see Position **2**). Hold for a 2 count. Release. Do 4 sets of 8 reps, each leg.

BENCH JUMPS

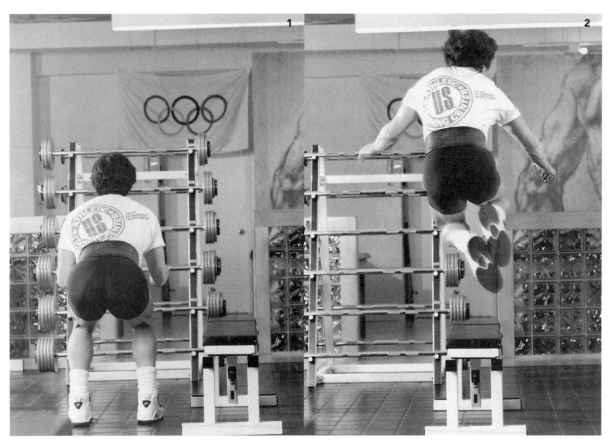

Assume the readiness position beside the free-weight bench (see Position **1**). Bend your knees and jump completely over bench—*sideways* (see Positions **2** and **3**). Then jump back. Do 5 sets of 5 reps.

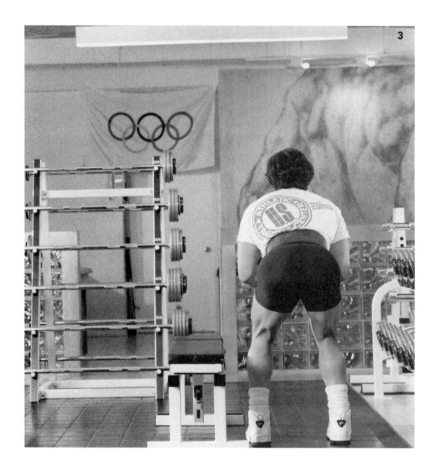

SPRINTS WITH RESISTANT TUBING

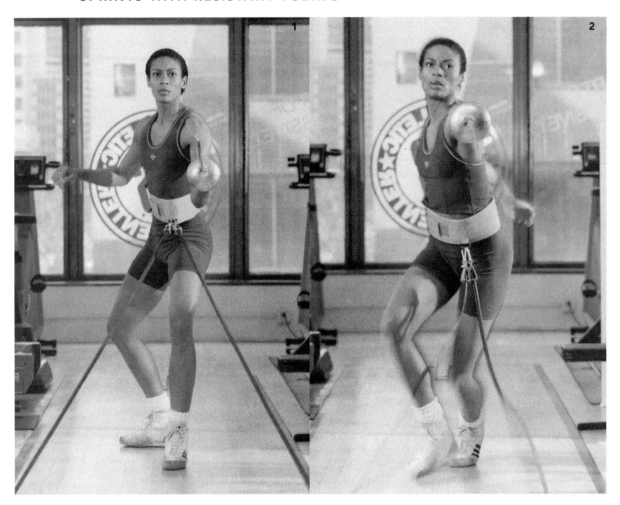

This is a pure fencing exercise called "fleché," and it's fun! Assume the fencing position (see Position **1**). Back up to stretch out the tubing, then do an explosive sprint forward (see Position **2**). Do about 6 paces, like a plane catapulted off an aircraft carrier. Do 5 sprints (with or without the sword!). The photos will give you an idea of the movement. Rest 30 seconds between sprints. Repeat 4 more times.

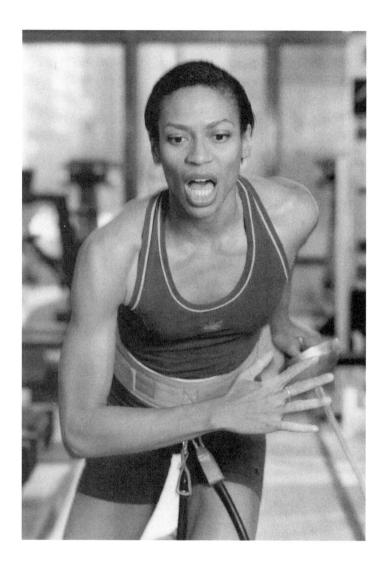

BOX JUMPS

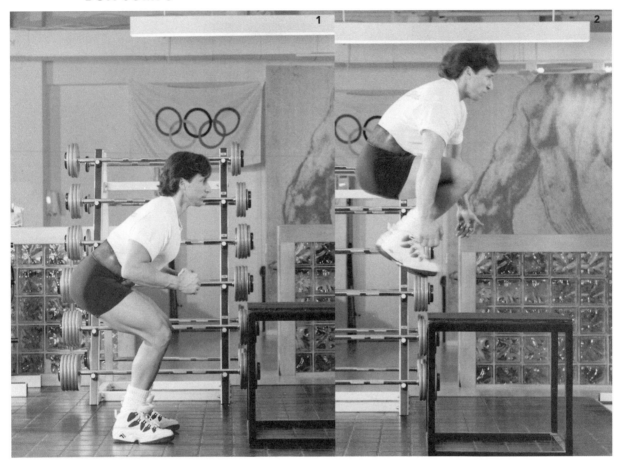

Assume the readiness position facing a sturdy 12-inch high box (see Position **1**). (You can graduate to 18- and 24-inch high boxes as you improve.) Leap atop the box (see Positions **2** and **3**). Then drop off backwards to Position **1**. Do 5 sets of 5 reps.

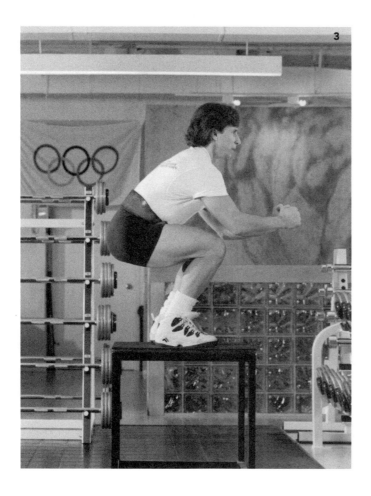

DEPTH JUMPS

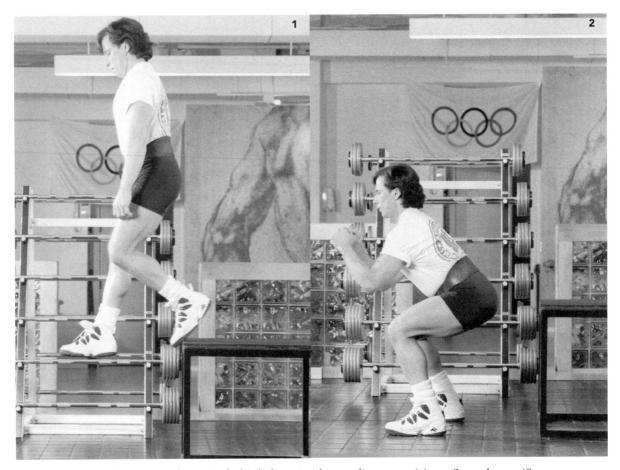

Stand on a sturdy 12-inch high box in the readiness position. Step down (See Position **1**) and land on floor with bent knees (see Position **2**). Then, from the readiness position, explode back upwards with a high-as-you-can-go jump (see Position **3**), landing in place. Do 5 sets of 5 reps.

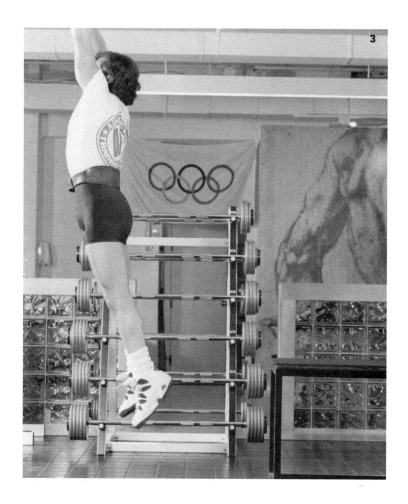

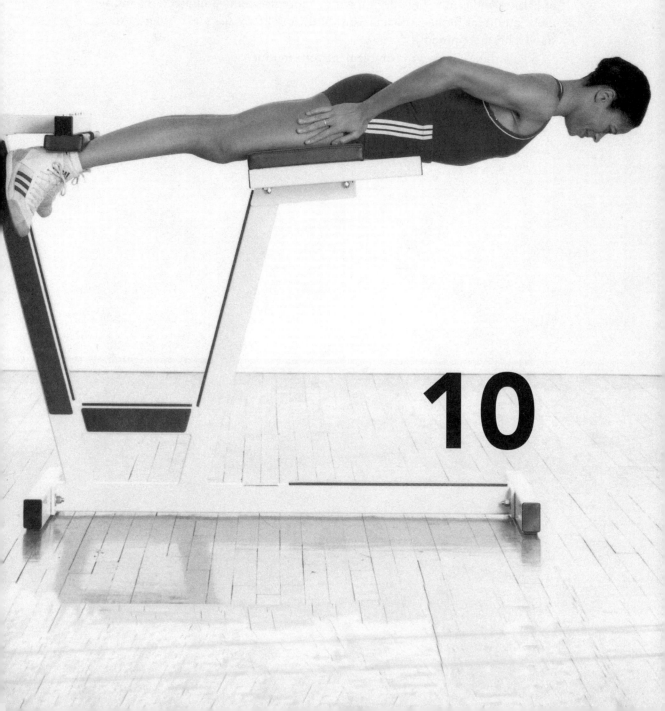

SPECIAL TRUNK AND ABDOMINAL STRENGTHENING EXERCISES

10

A trimmer, stronger stomach will give you better posture, improve your sense of balance and center, provide you with a more streamlined midsection, and—most important for us—enhance your butt. A tighter waist makes your butt stand a bit more proudly!

So use these exercises to complement your routine.

HANGING LEG RAISES

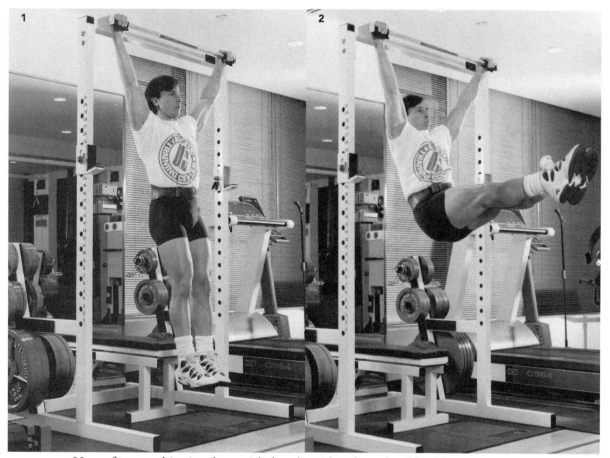

Hang from a chinning bar, with hands wider than shoulders (see Position **1**). Holding tightly to the bar, belly button pressed to spine, slowly raise legs until they are parallel to floor (see Position **2**). Pause briefly, and slowly lower legs. Do 5 sets of 5 reps. (This one is tough at first, but what results!)

Checkpoint for Leg Raises

Don't arch your back and no swinging! The movement begins with a pelvic tilt and your focus on lower abs to pull up your legs.

BENT KNEE RAISES IN STRAPS

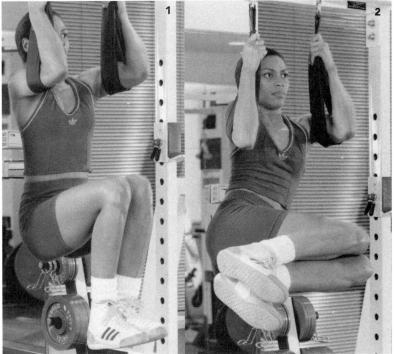

This one's a lot easier than the leg raises.

Insert arms in straps, and grasp the top of the strap. Extend your legs as you did in the Hanging Leg Raise, only this time bring knees up toward chest (see Position **1**), then lower slowly. Do 4 sets of 20 reps.

For a bent-knee diagonal (an invention of Mary's), bring knees toward chest, then lift legs to left, soles of feet facing wall (see Position **2**). Do 5 sets of 5 reps.

POP-UPS

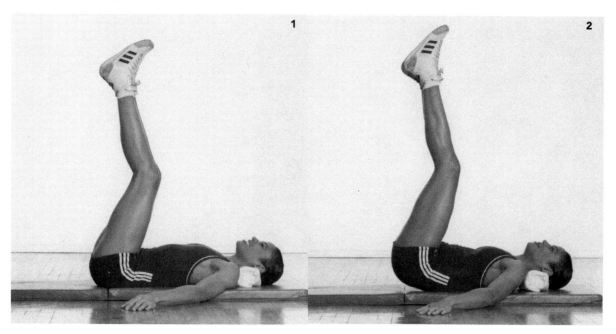

Lie on the mat, with legs extended, knees bent, and a rolled towel under your neck for support. Arms should be resting beside buttocks (see Position **1**). Lift the small of your back from the floor with a pelvic tilt (see Position **2**). Hold for a 2 count. Do 4 sets of 8 reps.

SIDE TO SIDES

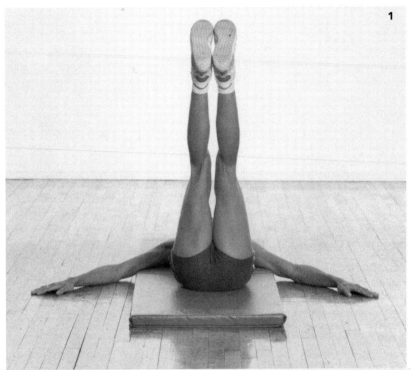

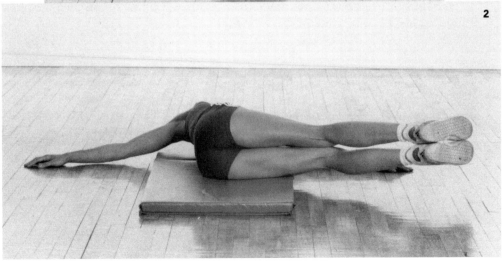

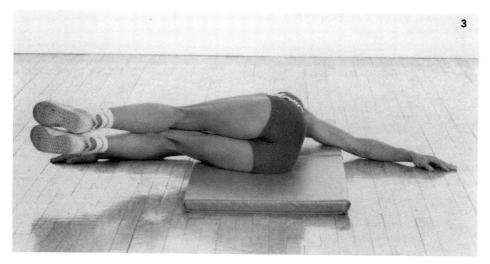

Lie on the mat, with your legs extended, knees bent, and a rolled towel under your neck. Hands should be outstretched, flat on the floor (see Position **1**). Turn legs slowly, from one side to the other, using your side trunk muscles to make the move, *not* your buttocks (see Positions **2** and **3**). This is a fantastic tire deflator. Do 5 sets of 5 reps.

MODIFIED STRAIGHT LEG RAISE

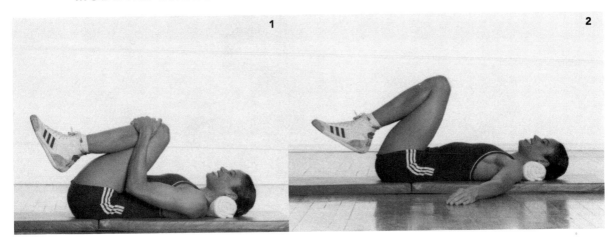

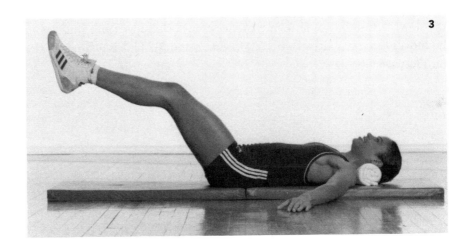

Lying on your back, start with your hands clasping knees toward chest, with a rolled towel under your neck for support. Keep belly button pressed to spine, and maintain pelvic tilt (Position **1**) Extend legs and lower them slowly, keeping lower back on floor while maintaining pelvic tilt (see Positions **2** and **3**). Bring knees back to chest and repeat. Do 5 sets of 5 reps.

SIMPLE CRUNCHES

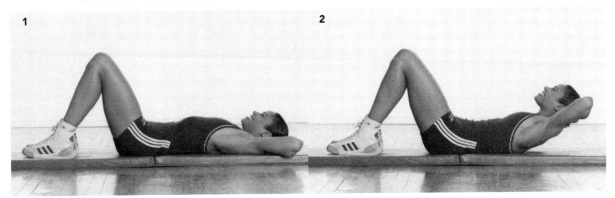

Lie on the mat, hands behind head, elbows out to the side (see Position **1**). Lift head and shoulders off the mat until your upper back is clear from floor (see Position **2**). Hold for a 2 count, slowly release. Keep belly button pressed toward spine, maintaining pelvic tilt. Do 4 sets of 15 to 50 reps.

CROSS SIT UP

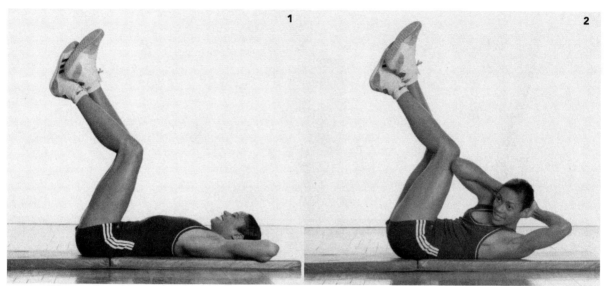

Lie on the mat, with hands behind head and legs extended, knees slightly bent, ankles crossed (see Position **1**). Lift right elbow to touch left knee (see Position **2**). Hold for a 2 count. Return to center and lower yourself to the floor. Repeat with left elbow to right knee. Hold for a 2 count, return to center and lower to floor. After each set, cross opposite ankles. Do 4 sets of 15 to 50 reps.

BACK EXTENSION

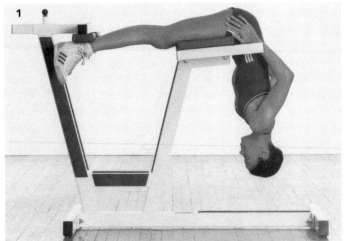

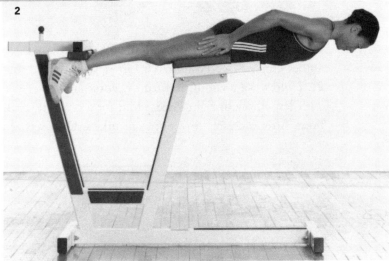

Lie on the back extension machine. Place hands on hips, belly button pressed toward spine (see Position **1**). Slowly rise up until your trunk is pulled parallel to the floor (see Position **2**). Hold for a 2 count. Lower slowly, then repeat. Keep buttocks and abs squeezed tightly throughout. Do 5 sets of 5 reps.

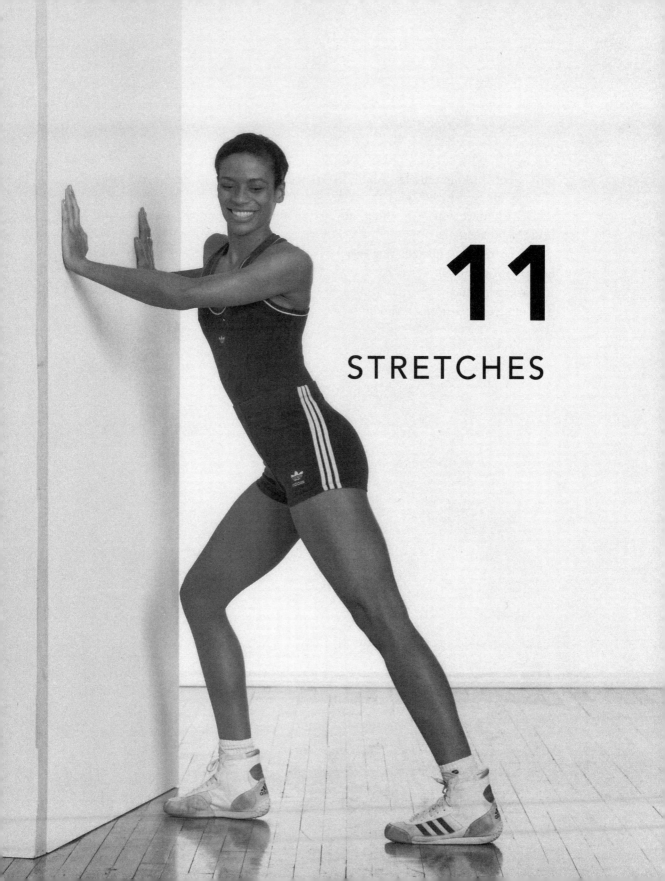

11
STRETCHES

Stretching is important. It keeps your muscles limber and loose. It helps heal those hard-working muscles. And it makes you feel terrific. Consider stretching as a way to reward your body for giving you 110 percent.

Don't bounce while stretching, just let the muscles pull slowly, gradually, and really feel that stretch.

After you've completed your exercises on any given day, be sure to give your body the stretching it deserves!

Also, continue with a controlled breathing pattern and never create more than moderate tension—it should be *relaxing*!

BEGINNER STRETCHES: HAMSTRINGS AND ADDUCTORS

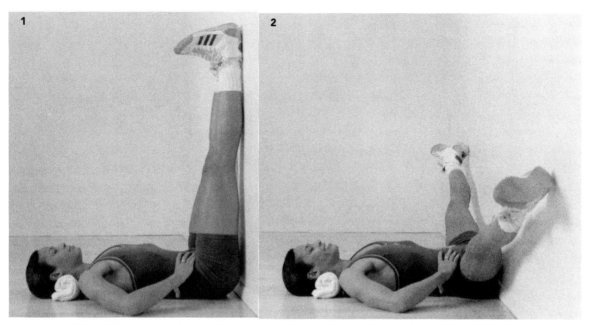

Lie with your back on the floor, and your buttocks on the wall, off the floor. Then sink back until your buttocks are on the floor. You've now settled into the correct position (see Position **1**). Lower your legs, toes flexed outward, to 9:15 position (see Position **2**). (Don't worry, you'll get closer to it with time.) Hold for 20 to 30 seconds.

QUAD

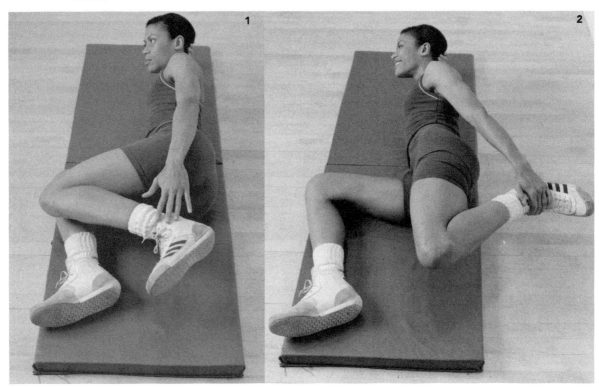

Rest your head on your right hand. Keep belly button pressed to spine, and hold abdominals tight, maintaining pelvic tilt throughout (see Position **1**). Grasp your left ankle with your left hand, and pull leg back and out, away from buttocks (see Position **2**). Hold for 30 seconds. Repeat for opposite side.

HAMSTRING

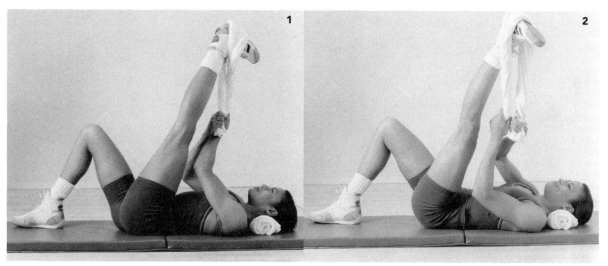

Lie on your back, with a rolled towel behind your neck and your right leg bent. Extend left leg. Drape another towel over heel and draw leg slowly toward body. You should feel moderate tension as you turn your entire leg in, rotating it in the hip socket (see Position **1**). Hold for 20 to 30 seconds. Release. Repeat, rotating leg out (see Position **2**). Hold for 20 to 30 seconds. You should also do this stretch without rotating the leg.

LOWER BACK

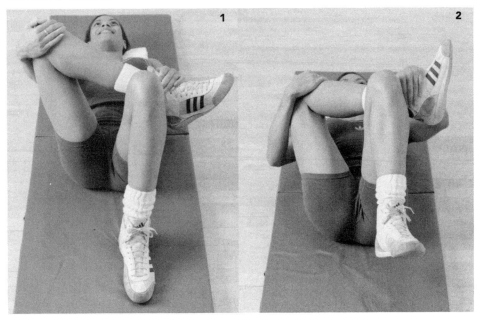

Lie flat on your back, with a rolled towel behind your neck. Hook your right foot behind your left knee (see Position **1**). Pull your right knee down with your right hand (see Position **2**). Hold for 20 to 30 seconds. Repeat for the opposite side.

CALF

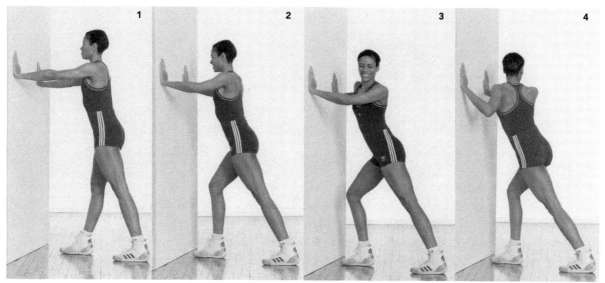

Stand facing a wall or table. Bring your left leg back, belly button to spine, and attempt a pelvic tilt (see Position **1**). Lean into the wall until you feel the stretch in your calf (see Position **2**). Keeping your front knee bent, back heel flat on floor, rotate hip slightly to left (see Position **3**). Return to the center, then rotate slightly to the right (see Position **4**). Return to center. Repeat for opposite side.

SPECIAL LOWER BACK

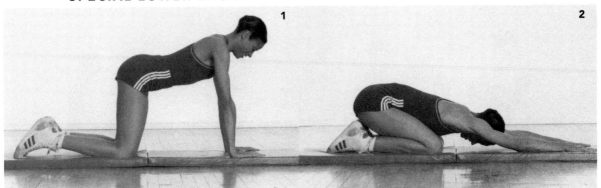

Get down on all fours (see Position **1**). Lean back until you're sitting on your heels, body forward, hands outstretched (see Position **2**). Concentrate on breathing in through your nose, out through your mouth. Feel the slow stretch. Relax. Relax some more. Relax *completely*. Hold for just as long as you feel like, 2 minutes or even 3.

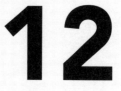

12

LITTLE THINGS
MEAN A LOT

Now that you've got your Gold Medal Butt, how can you keep it forever? Here are easy maintenance tips to protect your Gold Medal Butt against time and temptation.

1. Flex your Gold Medal Butt every chance you get. When you're sitting, *squeeze* your buttocks together. Actually lift your body an inch or more higher. It's easy to do 25 or 50 times during the day. But don't keep count—just do it whenever it occurs to you.

2. When you're walking, be aware of the glute that's pushing the opposite foot forward. Clutch it tight, to give your step an added bounce. Others won't notice, but you will. It makes walking a pleasure.

3. Walk and stand, always, with your belly button pressed toward your spine, just as you did during your exercises. Here's why that's so good for you: This simple belly button press activates your abdominal muscles right around your torso. The belly button press holds your tummy flat, and, most important of all, it holds your lower back in place. This simple trick eliminates the slump that can contribute to lower back pain.

4. Please, please don't gain weight. You've picked up so many good eating habits, and gotten rid of so many bad ones, what a shame if you let things go. Of course, once in a great while, when you've just had it with healthy eating, say right out loud "I'm going to pig out. Just this once, and to heck with the consequences!" Okay. Do it. Get it over with. But only one meal. Never two. Afterwards, you'll feel really guilty, and be glad you do. That's a light-hearted guilt that will nag you back on track. To counterattack, just cut back on your main meal the next day, or even skip it completely. It won't hurt you, and you'll drop any weight you may have added by indulging just once.

5. Take your favorite daily activity—walking, dancing, even shopping—and build little moves you learned in your Gold Medal Butt Program into it. This will keep you aware of the beautiful muscles you now own, and make you even more determined to keep them.

6. Choose any three exercises from these Gold Medal Butt forever maintenance moves, and do them for just ten minutes a day, three days a week. You'll never lose your shape.

Congratulations.

And may you always look this great—coming or going!

QUESTIONS THE DOUBTING THOMASES ASK MARY AND GARY

13

All These Skeptics Now Sport Gold Medal Butts!

Marga T.: I'm, scared. My backside is none too small as it is. Suppose your program makes it even bigger?!

Gary: Can't happen. You've hit upon another great thing about muscles. They don't make fat increase, they make it disappear. As you slip into the program, the six major muscles we're interested in can react in only three ways.

1. They have to tighten.
2. They will slim you.
3. They must lift your buttocks.

Now, is that good news, or what?

Jenny H.: I've never been much of an athlete. I'll never get the hang of it, and will probably do it all wrong.

Mary: Listen. I've always been an athlete. But all that exertion didn't get me a Gold Medal Butt. I didn't have one in high school, college, before or after my two kids were born. I won mine seven months ago, when I started following the program that Gary devised right here in our U.S. Athletic Training Center. Since then, I've helped lots of women win their Gold Medal Butts. Women of all kinds, from real tomboys to never-touch-the-stuff couch potatoes. And, while I can't prove it scientifically, my twenty-twenty eyesight tells me that the nonathletic women show even more dramatic changes than the sporty types. And I sure can prove that those women were much more ecstatic about their new behinds.

Colleen M.: With two kids, when would I find the time?

Gary: Oh, come on! Give it a try. Give it the time of, say, one of your soaps. In fact, do it while your watching your favorite TV show. Do it after the kids fall asleep. Better yet, let the older kids do it with you. They'll love it, and they'll get improved posture and balance in the bargain.

Rebecca R.: Look at me! I'm twenty-plus pounds overweight right now. Shouldn't I really diet that off first, so all that fat doesn't turn into muscle?

Mary: Rebecca—don't you dare diet first. What a mistake! You know why?

1. It won't be fun.
2. If you lose the weight, your butt'll still be flabby.
3. Your fat cannot, no matter what, turn into muscle.

Fat is fat. Period. So, forget dieting first. You get yourself right on this Gold Medal Butt Program. Three months down that slenderizing road, those fat-pounds will have been driven away; those six major muscles will be toning and strengthening and lifting your shape—you'll be showing off your Gold Medal Butt and you'll be eating better than ever. And that's a promise.

Kim W.: All right, tell me this. How come I haven't already got a Gold Medal Butt. I watch my weight, I do aerobics, I even jump rope!

Mary: Aha! But you're not doing these specialized, concentrated, pinpointed moves. There are dozens and dozens of muscles in your body that you can work to death, but only these six that we've isolated can affect your butt. And though the moves are simple, they simply aren't moves that happen in everyday activity. That's why they get such dramatic results. This program startles those powerful muscles into their new, compact, rounded shape. Just watch.

Nancy D.: I don't know. I've struggled with one plan, battled with another. None of them seem to—

Gary: Just stop right there! You're not alone. Lots of us are in the same boat. The stores are jammed with self-improvement sections, exercise miracles, aerobic menus. And most of them do work . . . for the dedicated and the long-term user. But here's the helpful, hopeful, result-filled difference: Once you jump into the Gold Medal Butt Program, you're taking aim at just one specific (though trouble-some) part of your anatomy. And luckily, scientifically, it happens to be a part that responds easily and dramatically to the proper, pinpointed, concentrated exercises. I'm talking about the one's we've developed, tested, and got our beautiful results

with. I know you've heard it all before. But nobody's ever worked with moves like this before. Except for fencers. And they're living proof the program works.
(P.S.: Nancy D. began and completed the program and she's got the Gold Medal Butt to prove it.)

Vivian S.: Here's what I always worry about. What if I can't keep up? It's been a long while since I really worked out or anything.

Mary: I hear you, Viv, but it's okay. These don't have to be speed drills. In fact, time isn't the most important factor at all. Much better for you to do the moves smoothly, while you concentrate your mind on the muscles you're exercising. And you don't have to understand anatomy to do that. You can feel these babies; and you'll just know they're starting to do the job.

Kelly P.: I never thought I'd be asking such a question, but I'd really hate to get too muscular.

Gary: And I'd hate to have you get too muscular. Let me repeat something about muscles. The ones we're strengthening in your Gold Medal Butt Program are being taught to tighten themselves, to tone themselves, to lift, lift, lift your buttocks. At the same time, they're shaping by contouring and curving. Your new butt is round, not muscle-bound.

Olivia J.: Somebody has to say it, so it might as well be me. Just how sore am I going to get, if you don't mind.

Mary: Speaking as America's foremost coward when it comes to pain, let me say this: That cynical slogan "no pain—no gain" is baloney. Now let me say this: The first couple of days you'll feel a little stiffness, a little soreness, but nothing bad, really. Here's a funny thing about soreness as opposed to pain. The soreness you'll feel here is, well, satisfying. It's dull and low-level. (You feel it because these unaccustomed moves, like all exercise, create tiny, microscopic tears where the tendons and ligaments join the muscle. In repairing these tiny tears, your body makes those muscles stronger. Nice, huh?) Pain, on the other hand, is a sharp, warning sensation that accompanies actual injury. It's highly unlikely that you'll encounter pain during these carefully selected moves, but if you should, stop the exercise. And if pain persists, see your physician.

Elaine C.: I should be so lucky, but I've heard of people who work out but don't lose weight, even though they look better and drop a couple of sizes.

Gary: Not only can that happen, it probably will happen to you. It means you're on your way to your Gold Medal Butt. Here's what's going down there. As you get into your program, your moves are going to be driving away fat; and at the same time adding size to your muscle. And muscle weighs more than fat, even though it takes up significantly less space. So your shadow will be shrinking long before your scale notices a damn thing. Soon enough, though, you'll start dropping those pounds, too. Because your new muscles eat up more calories than fat. (That's why you can eat so well on the program.)

The Ten Commandments

According to Mary and Gary

---

1. Keep your belly button pressed toward your spine. This automatically holds your abdominals tight and protects your lower back.

2. Whenever you are raising or lowering your body, let your effort drive (or *push*) through your heels. This both protects the knees and develops the butt.

3. Always place a rolled up towel (about 4 inches in diameter) behind your neck on all exercises that involve lying on the floor. The support provided decreases cervical pressure and compression.

4. Remember that free weights have this advantage over machines: Because they're dead weight, they must be moved. This increases tension and improves development. It also adds balance and coordination to the exercise, helping to increase its effectiveness.

5. Concentrate on *feeling* the muscle you're working on. Isolate it, feel it, squeeze it. Become one with your muscle.

6. Tolerate *no* pain, ever, in your joints when exercising. If you do experience pain, check your technique. Did you warm up? Try decreasing the weight you're using or decreasing the range of motion. Stretch to relieve tightness. (If pain persists, see your physician.)

7. Obey the training variables as specified in each of the exercises of the program:

   Intensity (poundage or weights)
   Duration (sets)
   Frequency (repetitions)
   Never increase more than one variable
   Never increase any variable more than 10 percent per week

8. Make the most of the variables in the exercise program:

Rest periods
Varying exercises
Types of workouts (intersperse home workouts with gym programs)

9. During each day do some isometrics: for example, exert against an unmovable object or tense one buttock against the other, hold 5 to 6 seconds. Or try to press thighs together while holding them apart with your hands. Tough, but a fast, effective exercise.

10. Drink water before you work out. While you work out. After you work out. *Don't* wait till you're thirsty. Drink!

WRITE TO US

If you have any questions or comments,
please drop us a line at:

Gary Guerriero and Mary Leonard
c/o U.S. Athletic Training Center
515 Madison Avenue
New York, NY 10022